1992

The Challenge

for States

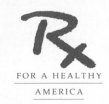

FOR A HEALTHY
AMERICA

THE NATIONAL GOVERNORS' ASSOCIATION, founded in 1908 as the National Governors' Conference, is the instrument through which the nation's Governors collectively influence the development and implementation of national policy and apply creative leadership to state issues. The association's members are the Governors of the fifty states, the commonwealths of the Northern Mariana Islands and Puerto Rico, and the territories of American Samoa, Guam, and the Virgin Islands.

The association has seven standing committees on major issues: Agriculture and Rural Development, Economic Development and Technological Innovation, Energy and Environment, Human Resources, International Trade and Foreign Relations, Justice and Public Safety, and Transportation, Commerce, and Communications. Subcommittees and task forces that focus on principal concerns of the Governors operate within this framework.

The association works closely with the administration and Congress on state-federal policy issues from its offices in the Hall of the States in Washington, D.C. The association serves as a vehicle for sharing knowledge of innovative programs among the states and provides technical assistance and consultant services to Governors on a wide range of management and policy issues. The Center for Policy Research serves the Governors by undertaking demonstration projects and providing anticipatory research on important policy issues.

Funding for this report was provided in part by the Pew Charitable Trusts.

Publication design by Genovese Coustenis Design.

Photograph by Susie Fitzhugh.

Printed on recycled paper.

ISBN 1-55877-125-5

Contents

Foreword

A healthy America. That is the challenge and the opportunity that lies before us.

The National Governors' Association Task Force on Health Care has spent the past year considering ways to ensure that every American has access to and can afford the care he or she needs to be healthy.

The challenge is great. This nation faces one of its most critical domestic crises ever. The country's health care systems are in serious trouble. Millions of citizens lack access to basic medical care. Businesses and governments face double-digit increases in employee insurance premiums. Hospitals and clinics are at risk of closing and leaving some communities without adequate medical resources. Meanwhile, governments strain merely to respond with stopgap measures.

The choices we have before us have never been more complex. States face the most difficult fiscal crisis of the decade. There isn't enough revenue to meet current program demands, let alone take on pressing social needs. Yet as health care devours even greater shares of our state budgets and more citizens go without needed care, something clearly needs to be done.

A year of work on this issue has convinced us that there are no short, quick, painless answers. But after a national conference, regional hearings, and extensive outreach to those whose lives are touched by the health care system, we firmly believe that solutions are possible and that states are well positioned to find them.

States are major purchasers of health care coverage for their employees; regulators and licensors of both medical care providers and medical care facilities; regulators of the insurance industry; and financiers of health care through Medicaid and their public health programs.

The nation's Governors are charting a course toward a comprehensive national health care system. A consensus on the shape of such a system does not yet exist. We are beginning by focusing our attention on what states can do now.

This is a critical step because while there are many theories about health care reform, most of them are untested. Trying and evaluating these programs will help give us the concrete data we need to undertake wide-scale reform. States already are developing and testing innovative solutions. Through information gathering, sharing, and debate, Governors hope to expand the strategies they use to tackle difficult health care issues. That forum will include an open and informed exchange of ideas with members of the business, medical, and academic communities.

All Governors may not agree with everything in this report. Consensus is not the intent. As each state analyzes its own problems, its own people, and its own strengths, choices will be made about the approaches that are most appropriate.

Governors want to build a consensus that will lead to meaningful reform. The innovation and experimentation outlined in these pages can help move us toward affordable and appropriate health care for all Americans.

Members of the NGA Task Force on Health Care

Booth Gardner, Chairman
Governor of Washington
Chairman, National Governors' Association

Bill Clinton, Vice Chairman
Governor of Arkansas

Michael N. Castle, Vice Chairman
Governor of Delaware

John Ashcroft
Governor of Missouri, *Ex Officio*

John R. McKernan Jr.
Governor of Maine
Chair, Committee on Human Resources

Pete Wilson
Governor of California

Lowell P. Weicker Jr.
Governor of Connecticut

Lawton Chiles
Governor of Florida

John Waihee
Governor of Hawaii

Terry E. Branstad
Governor of Iowa

Buddy Roemer
Governor of Louisiana

John Engler
Governor of Michigan

Jim Florio
Governor of New Jersey

Carroll A. Campbell Jr.
Governor of South Carolina

Ann W. Richards
Governor of Texas

Executive Summary

The health of a nation depends on the health of its people. The Governors share a vision of an America in which all people can attain a level of health that will permit them to lead socially and economically productive lives. But for that vision to become reality, purposeful change must occur, and Governors can do much to pave the way.

Clearly, the nation's health care system is in trouble. The system costs too much and provides too little. Moreover, there are increasing questions about the value of what is purchased.

The cost statistics are familiar. Total health spending has grown from less than 6 percent of the gross national product (GNP) in 1960 to about 12 percent in 1990. It is projected to reach 17 percent of GNP by the year 2000, and 37 percent of GNP by the year 2030. Similarly, state spending has increased at exponential rates. States currently spend more than 20 percent of their budgets on health. Medicaid spending alone has grown by 18 percent in 1990, far outpacing the growth of state economies.

Despite the extraordinary amount spent on health care, access to health insurance and health care is uneven. Roughly 34 million nonelderly Americans have no health coverage at all. Human potential is being wasted needlessly as an increasing number of citizens find even routine preventive and primary care beyond their reach.

Governors realize that while the cost and access statistics are grim, attention to the financing and delivery of medical care alone will not achieve the goal of a healthy America. For health is also a consequence of environment, lifestyle, education, and income.

Governors have taken and will continue to assume significant responsibility for the policies, programs, and resources to address these factors. Yet precious resources that Governors want to invest in education, housing, nutrition, and family support are being consumed by the spiraling costs of medical care.

WHAT CAN GOVERNORS DO?

While there is growing consensus on the nature and extent of the health care problems confronting the nation, there is little consensus on the solutions. That consensus can be forged based on the results of aggressive and creative state-based reforms of the system.

The Governors believe a way to achieve national consensus is to develop comprehensive, statewide health care reforms that maximize preventive and public health programs and experiment with medical care payment programs to reduce overall medical costs.

Why states? First, because Governors have a significant number of important policy levers at their command. They not only are major purchasers of care, but also regulate insurance, license health care professionals and institutions, allocate capital resources, and deliver services.

Further, states are at once both large enough to leverage the development of an effective health care market and small enough to organize a health care delivery system that is close to the people and meets the unique needs of different populations.

Finally, any national consensus on health care reform that emerges will need to be based on state administration of the system to ensure an appropriate service delivery system sensitive to local needs.

HOW CAN THIS REPORT HELP?

This report is premised on the belief that it will be some years before national consensus is reached about how best to reform the nation's health care system. It further assumes that no Governor can afford to wait for national consensus before taking action.

The report, therefore, not only raises and explores the significant problems in the health care system, but also provides both incremental, concrete options and bold, alternative strategies that states can employ to:

Reorient the Health Care System Toward Preventive and Primary Care Services.
A health care system that focuses on promoting and maintaining health rather than treating sickness rests on a foundation of providing systematic and routine preventive and primary care services to everyone. Positive changes in health status are possible if effective preventive and primary care services are adopted at the community and provider level. States can be active catalysts for a reorientation of the health system toward preventive and primary care services. Examples of state strategies include:

✦ Fostering community-based services;

✦ Employing creative ways to use current resources such as local public health departments and schools to ensure access to basic services;

✦ Focusing the state investment in the education of health professionals on preventive and primary care through expanded training opportunities, and extending the use of mid-level practitioners;

✦ Mandating preventive and primary coverage in health insurance benefit packages; and

✦ Improving current preventive and primary care practices in state programs such as the Medicaid Early and Periodic Screening, Diagnostic, and Treatment (EPSDT) program.

Develop Ways to Both Encourage and Assist Businesses in Finding Affordable Health Insurance for Their Employees, and to Stabilize Coverage for Employees Already Receiving Health Insurance.
Of the estimated 34.4 million nonelderly Americans without health insurance, more than 80 percent are either workers or their dependents. Access to the health care system in the United States generally is through employer-based health insurance coverage, but the significant number of working uninsured attests to the problems employers face in finding affordable insurance. This is especially true for small businesses that are less likely to offer coverage to their employees.

There are a number of strategies states can initiate to address this problem of the working uninsured. These include:

✦ Requiring employers to offer health coverage under the employer-based health insurance system;

✦ Implementing mechanisms to reduce health insurance costs, including targeting benefits, reducing the cost of health insurance premiums, directly subsidizing premium costs (employer tax credits, for example) and indirectly subsidizing the cost of insurance;

✦ Directly financing the cost of care by leveraging public funds like Medicaid on behalf of uninsured workers; and

✦ Ensuring that the insurance market functions effectively.

Identify the Unique Needs of the Disparate Populations Who Comprise the Nonworking Uninsured and Develop Systems of Care to Address These Needs.
Medicaid was created to respond to the problems of specific vulnerable populations. However, it has become a complex program that does not always meet the needs of those for whom it was intended. Medicaid also currently cannot be deemed a comprehensive approach to provide health coverage to the nonworking population. The states have an enormous investment in Medicaid and other state programs to assist vulnerable populations and must use these resources wisely to improve access for large numbers of individuals who are without any coverage at all.

Options available to the states include:

✦ Building on the existing Medicaid program (through Medicaid buy-ins, for example);

✦ Using insurance subsidies to assist selected populations to secure health coverage (for example, through high-risk pools);

✦ Establishing universal coverage for selected populations (children, for example);

✦ Providing public catastrophic insurance for high-expense illnesses;

✦ Directly funding health services rather than making changes in health insurance coverage; and

✦ Enhancing voluntary efforts by providers to provide care for those in need.

Make Better Use of Incremental Cost Control Strategies That Currently Are Available to Every Governor.

While ensuring access to health services is critical, it cannot be done in the absence of cost control strategies. Because states are the the nation's second largest purchaser of health services, they have a vested interest in exercising all means at their command to control costs. There are several generic strategies states can employ to control the cost of health care incrementally. These include:

✦ Using managed care strategies aggressively;

✦ Leveraging the state's buying power in the health care system to garner substantial discounts;

✦ Reducing the impact of cost shifting through such means as provider taxes and revenue pooling arrangements; and

✦ Making better use of existing regulatory cost containment tools, including certificate of need, hospital rate setting, and malpractice reforms.

Take Bold Steps to Implement Major Structural Changes in the Health Care System at the State Level to Significantly Check the Rise in Health Care Costs.

Incremental cost control strategies hold some promise for controlling costs in the short run, but major structural changes are needed if costs are to be controlled in the long run. In essence, there are two polar positions regarding health care resource allocation—a market-oriented approach or a public allocation approach.

Regardless of which approach is adopted, each constitutes major structural change in the way health care is financed and each promises to reduce the cost of health care.

To move toward a more market-oriented strategy, there are a series of actions a state would need to take. These actions address the major causes of failure in the health care market—lack of information, the role of insurance in generating unnecessary demand for health care and decreasing price consciousness, barriers to entry for providers, and health insurance industry practices.

The public allocation approach generally eschews the market as the way to allocate health care resources. It requires greater intervention on the part of state government. Basically two alternatives are possible—an all-payor approach and a single-payor approach. The all-payor approach centralizes health care payment decisions in a single quasi-public agency that negotiates payments between providers and purchasers. This approach retains financing from multiple payors. The single-payor approach, which funnels all financing and payments through a single source, has not been implemented in the United States, though there are several models of both tax-based and social insurance-based systems in Europe.

Seize the Opportunity to Move Beyond the Current System to Develop a Financing and Service Delivery System That Provides Access to All at Affordable Prices.

Gaps in access to coverage and escalating costs require fundamental change in the current health care system in the United States. The basic decision about structural reform is in essence a decision about the respective roles and responsibilities of the private and public sectors. The direction a Governor takes will depend on his or her beliefs about the nature of health care and how resources are to be allocated. Three possible approaches that might be taken are:

✦ Creating a single private system using public funds as a source of subsidies and reinsurance;

✦ Moving away from the employer-based health insurance system by using other means to group people and collect funds; and

✦ Publicly financing basic health care and using private insurance for catastrophic coverage.

This report is not intended to be a statistical status report of the health care system or a textbook for health policymakers. It is intended to encourage consideration of the fundamental questions that must be addressed in any successful health care reform strategy. It provides both information based on successful state experience and a conceptual framework for moving beyond what has already been tried.

The report asks Governors and other state policymakers to think about the ways they currently "do business" in health care and suggests changes that could be implemented to provide wider coverage to more people at affordable prices.

Several key points, which need to be considered by all states interested in significant reform, emerged in the report.

✦ There is a real need to systematically provide the public with information about health care. States must do a better job of ensuring that citizens have access to information about the availability, cost, and quality of medical care.

✦ There clearly is too much administrative waste in the system. Whether it is in the marketing of insurance, the multiplicity of overlapping utilization controls, or the complexity of billing and payment procedures, states must look for ways to reduce administrative overhead.

✦ Health care services need to be evaluated against appropriate standards to ensure that people are receiving effective health care services.

✦ The dysfunctional state of the small business health insurance market must be addressed.

✦ Effective and efficient community-based services must be integrated into a state's health care financing and administrative structure.

✦ Malpractice must be addressed through tort reform, alternative dispute resolution, and/or the application of practice guidelines as a defensible standard.

✦ Careful consideration must be given to the needs of the poor, the working uninsured, and people with special needs to ensure that basic health care services are available to them. This probably will require rethinking the financing, benefits, and coverage of public programs.

✦ While a number of the incremental cost control strategies available to states will make some marginal differences in costs, real cost containment will require more dramatic, structural changes in the financing of care.

✦ There must be a shared commitment among states, the federal government, businesses, health care providers, insurers, and consumers to work together to achieve an equitable system for financing and delivering health care services.

WHY SHOULD GOVERNORS SEIZE THE OPPORTUNITY?

Reforming the health care system is the most complex, divisive, and politically explosive domestic challenge confronting the nation.

Effecting change, even at the state level, will require extraordinary political will, vigorous leadership, risk taking, and the ability to marshal unlikely coalitions of powerful interested parties.

It will require time, concerted effort, and a willingness to invest resources up front in the expectation of a future reward.

So why try? Because the nation simply cannot continue to spend vast sums of money shoring up a system that leaves out increasing numbers of people. America cannot afford either the human or the economic waste.

Governors must solicit the active participation of their communities—businesses, labor groups, providers, insurers, and people throughout the state—to create change.

Fear of change must not impede the effort. A more efficient system may be able to provide universal access without added costs and with less microregulation. Reform should not be feared. In fact, the challenges represent an exciting opportunity for all those in the system.

The costs of inaction are high. The nation cannot afford to leave the current health care system as it is. Without significant change at the state level, Governors increasingly will be faced with spiraling costs that rob them of the freedom and flexibility to invest in other issues that are vital for a healthy citizenry and a productive economy. If steps are not taken now to build a real health care system, too many children will continue to come to school unprepared to learn, too many adolescents will continue to face serious but preventable health problems, and too many adults will be prevented from leading full and productive lives.

If health care systems are a reflection of societal values, it is time to make the U.S. system reflect the generosity and caring that are so intrinsic to the nation's history and values. Through innovation and experimentation, Governors can seize the opportunity to develop a health care financing and service delivery system that provides access to all at affordable prices.

The Challenge

SUMMARY Today the spiraling cost of health care is consuming precious resources that are required for other basic needs such as education, housing, nutrition, and family support. Yet, not only do increasing numbers of people not have financial access to care through insurance or public programs, but also there is concern that the nation is not buying a healthier America.

The health care system is a patchwork of multiple public and private financing mechanisms, each with its own rules for eligibility, payment, and coverage. Rather than working cooperatively, the public and private sectors compete, each protecting its own interests and each trying to reduce its own risks and costs. As a result, there are gaps in coverage, duplication of effort, and high administrative costs.

Governors control a number of policy levers that can be used to improve access, ensure quality, and control costs. These include educating and certifying providers, regulating insurers, and providing employee benefits. Governors cannot afford to wait for a national consensus before undertaking serious reform. The costs of inaction are too high.

WHAT IS THE GOVERNORS' VISION?

In 1977 the United States and other member countries of the World Health Organization asserted that health is a fundamental human right. The participating nations agreed on a major objective for government: that all people attain a level of health that will permit them to lead socially and economically productive lives by the year 2000.

The nation's Governors share this vision. But attention to the financing and delivery of medical care alone will not achieve the goal. For health is also a consequence of environment, genetic endowment, lifestyle, education, and income.

Governors are in a unique position to focus attention on health and to communicate to the public that medical care is just one of the many factors affecting health. They have significant responsibility for the policies, pro-

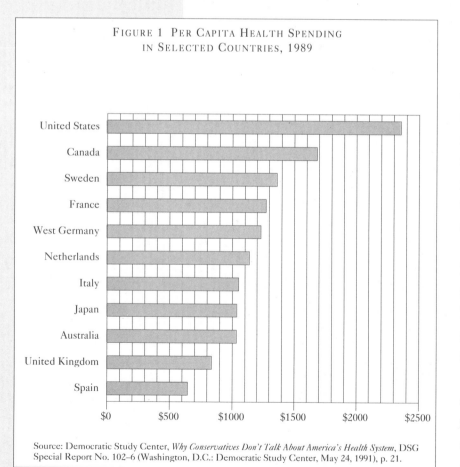

FIGURE 1 PER CAPITA HEALTH SPENDING IN SELECTED COUNTRIES, 1989

Source: Democratic Study Center, *Why Conservatives Don't Talk About America's Health System*, DSG Special Report No. 102–6 (Washington, D.C.: Democratic Study Center, May 24, 1991), p. 21.

grams, and resources to address these factors. Yet precious resources that could be invested in education, housing, nutrition, and family support are being consumed by the spiraling costs of health care, which are increasing at a rate exceeding general inflation. Moreover, access for many citizens is compromised; health status indicators are becoming poorer; and suspicion is growing that the nation's investment in medical care is not always producing effective outcomes.

WHAT IS THE PROBLEM?

The cost statistics are familiar:

✦ Total U.S. health spending has grown from less than 6 percent of the gross national product (GNP) in 1960 to about 12 percent of GNP in 1990. It currently is projected to reach 17 percent of GNP by the year 2000, and 37 percent of GNP by the year 2030.[1]

✦ Per capita health care costs in the United States are the highest in the world (see Figure 1).

✦ Price increases for medical care consistently outpace those for other commodities (see Figure 2).

✦ Health benefit costs now consume more than 25 percent of a firm's profits.[2]

✦ Personal out-of-pocket spending for health services continues to rise as a percentage of total spending for health. At the same time, most families have seen their incomes decline, in relative terms, during the past decade.[3]

Comparable figures suggest that the situation for states is no different:

✦ States currently spend more than 20 percent of their budgets on health.[4]

✦ Total health spending in the states increased dramatically between 1980 and 1990, as did per capita health spending. This level of spending is expected to continue between 1990 and 2000 (see Table 1).

✦ Medicaid expenditures grew by 18 percent in 1990, far outpacing the growth of state economies. This program has become the fastest growing item in many state budgets, absorbing more than 50 percent of revenue growth in some states.[5]

The level of expenditures alone would not be sufficient cause for concern if the resources were producing substantive health benefits. But the evidence suggests that this is not the case.

Despite the extraordinary amount of money spent, access to health insurance and care is uneven at best. Roughly 16 percent of the nonelderly have no health insurance.[6] Even more have inadequate access to routine preventive and primary care services. And, while being uninsured does not necessarily mean that one cannot receive medical care, those who are uninsured or underinsured are more likely to wait to seek care until a medical crisis sends them to the most expensive setting to receive care. And being insured does not guarantee access to care.

Health insurance is not the only factor that determines whether people actually have access to health services. Access depends on an effective delivery system, so issues such as adequate funding of public health services, the transportation needs of poor and rural citizens, outreach efforts to help people use health care services more effectively, and the careful screening and licensing of health care personnel and facilities are important.

CAUSES OF THE
COST SPIRAL

Many variables drive health care spending, including:

Demographic changes;

General inflation;

Increased individual and societal expectations;

Changes in underlying disease patterns;

Technological advances;

Changes in the volume and intensity of services;

Malpractice premiums and defensive medicine; and

The nature of the health care system.

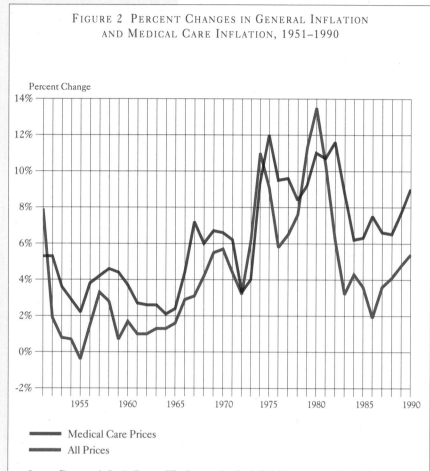

FIGURE 2 PERCENT CHANGES IN GENERAL INFLATION
AND MEDICAL CARE INFLATION, 1951–1990

Percent Change

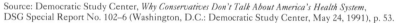
━━━ Medical Care Prices
━━━ All Prices

Source: Democratic Study Center, *Why Conservatives Don't Talk About America's Health System,*
DSG Special Report No. 102–6 (Washington, D.C.: Democratic Study Center, May 24, 1991), p. 53.

Real per capita health expenditures have risen dramatically and far outpace the per capita expenditures of all the United States' major industrialized trading partners. But is the nation buying a healthier citizenry? By several measures, U.S. health status is not conspicuously superior, and by some measures, it is clearly inferior. Canada, Germany, Great Britain, and Japan spend substantially less on health per capita and as a percentage of GNP, but these countries have lower infant mortality rates, lower maternal mortality rates, lower mortality rates for low-risk and moderate-risk surgery, and higher life expectancies for both men and women (see Figure 3).

Further, health status indicators in the United States are getting worse. Several long-defeated diseases—including tuberculosis, measles, and rabies—are now staging a comeback.[7] New challenges such as AIDS offer convincing evidence that the health care system is unable to cope.

Clearly, cost, access, and quality concerns remind all of the unacceptability of the current health care system. But the nation cannot be so single-minded in its pursuit of the perfect health care system that it ignores or forgets other factors influencing health. Moreover, while concerns about financial access have been the central focus of the public policy debate, efforts to reduce the rate of increase of health care costs and to use resources more effectively and efficiently must be pursued just as vigorously.

HOW DID THE CURRENT SYSTEM EVOLVE?

As the nation seeks to construct a system that is effective, efficient, and equitable for all Americans by the twenty-first century, it is important to understand how the U.S. health care system has evolved to put the current system into context and, perhaps, to learn the lessons of history.

The current health care system evolved in two distinct phases in the twentieth century. From the end of World War II through the 1960s, the nation's health care system witnessed phenomenal growth. During this period many Americans gained health insurance coverage for an ever increasing array of medical and health services. In contrast, since the 1970s there have been major efforts to control and constrain growth, albeit unsuccessfully.[8]

World War II Through the 1960s

The current health care system took root in the rapid growth of employer-based health insurance after World War II. The passage of the Medicare and Medicaid programs in 1965 became the public insurance models for the elderly, poor, and unemployed.

From the end of World War II through the 1960s, several major trends contributed to the development of today's health care system:

◆ Employers began to offer health insurance as a way to retain employees.

◆ Union representation of employees grew rapidly, and collective bargaining for health and medical benefits was legitimized by the Supreme Court.

◆ The United States enjoyed a period of great economic growth, with ample resources for medical care.

◆ There was tremendous growth in medical research, which led to greater specialization in the medical profession, a focus on curing specific diseases such as polio, and the extension of medical care to include mental health.

While health insurance was employer-based, it was structured on individual relationships. Insurance did not invade the physician-patient relationship. Insurers reimbursed the individual for medical services, and the individual paid the physician or hospital. In this early period, services were not an issue. Insurers paid for medical services based on physician authorization.

As private employer-based health insurance grew, greatly expanded financial resources were available for medical research. As new technologies and therapies were discovered, they were made available to physicians, hospitals, and the general public. In

TABLE 1 PER CAPITA HEALTH SPENDING (IN 1990 DOLLARS)							
STATE	1980	1990	2000	STATE	1980	1990	2000
Alabama	1,466	2,286	3,381	Montana	1,363	2,059	3,046
Alaska	1,461	2,367	3,504	Nebraska	1,612	2,452	3,625
Arizona	1,345	2,211	3,271	Nevada	1,759	2,757	4,077
Arkansas	1,339	1,944	2,875	New Hampshire	1,290	1,981	2,929
California	1,881	2,894	4,280	New Jersey	1,475	2,224	3,287
Colorado	1,580	2,415	3,573	New Mexico	1,128	1,792	2,651
Connecticut	1,821	2,699	3,989	New York	1,994	2,818	4,166
Delaware	1,523	2,268	3,355	North Carolina	1,226	1,833	2,711
District of Columbia	1,968	2,586	3,824	North Dakota	1,691	2,661	3,934
Florida	1,526	2,427	3,589	Ohio	1,648	2,493	3,684
Georgia	1,401	2,072	3,065	Oklahoma	1,437	2,139	3,164
Hawaii	1,575	2,469	3,653	Oregon	1,491	2,312	3,420
Idaho	1,123	1,726	2,554	Pennsylvania	1,620	2,536	3,747
Illinois	1,734	2,619	3,870	Rhode Island	1,878	2,707	4,000
Indiana	1,458	2,201	3,253	South Carolina	1,120	1,689	2,498
Iowa	1,575	2,351	3,474	South Dakota	1,510	2,322	3,431
Kansas	1,677	2,548	3,765	Tennessee	1,510	2,262	3,345
Kentucky	1,278	1,875	2,773	Texas	1,451	2,192	3,242
Louisiana	1,491	2,185	3,232	Utah	1,175	1,784	2,641
Maine	1,380	2,175	3,215	Vermont	1,293	1,956	2,892
Maryland	1,651	2,436	3,602	Virginia	1,369	2,076	3,071
Massachusetts	2,037	3,031	4,479	Washington	1,474	2,311	3,418
Michigan	1,740	2,569	3,797	West Virginia	1,337	2,088	3,089
Minnesota	1,761	2,480	3,667	Wisconsin	1,740	2,449	3,619
Mississippi	1,204	1,751	2,590	Wyoming	1,133	1,756	2,598
Missouri	1,639	2,568	3,795	**TOTAL**	**1,612**	**2,425**	**3,584**

Note: Figures for 2000 are estimates using the Health Benefits Simulation Model.
Source: Lewin/ICF, 1991.

this expansionary environment, technological advances moved quickly from the development phase to health care services paid for by private insurance.

The unbridled growth extended through the early 1960s and increased with the enactment of Medicare and Medicaid in 1965. These two government programs were intended to make health care coverage available to those who were not in the labor force and thus unable to get health insurance through the workplace. Medicare covered hospital and physician services for the elderly and disabled. Medicaid provided coverage to

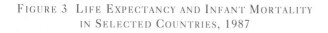

FIGURE 3 LIFE EXPECTANCY AND INFANT MORTALITY
IN SELECTED COUNTRIES, 1987

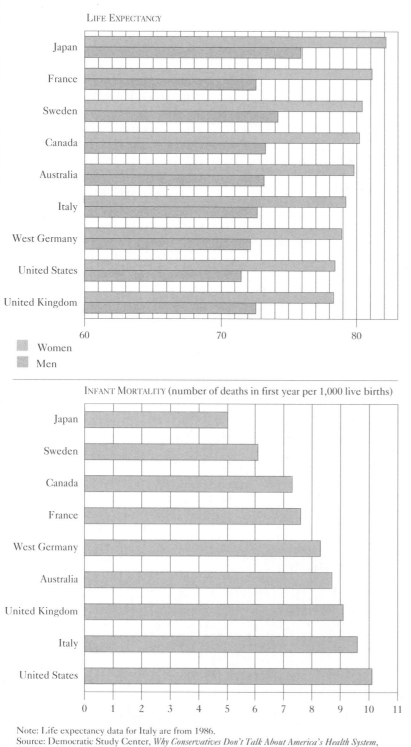

Note: Life expectancy data for Italy are from 1986.
Source: Democratic Study Center, *Why Conservatives Don't Talk About America's Health System*, DSG Special Report No. 102–6 (Washington, D.C.: Democratic Study Center, May 24, 1991), p. 26.

certain categories of the nonworking poor, primarily those eligible for income maintenance payments. Initially, there was little concern about the services and costs of these programs. Services and payment were piggybacked on the private employer-based insurance system.

The growth in the number of people with access to public and private health insurance was phenomenal during this period. In 1940 about 12 million people had private insurance coverage. By 1975 about 178 million people were covered through private health insurance, with an additional 47 million covered by Medicare and Medicaid.[9]

The 1970s to 1990s

The growth in health care expenditures became a major issue in the 1970s. A series of major legislative proposals were introduced to reform health care generally, and to address cost containment specifically. Although none were enacted, a number of incremental changes were adopted.

Efforts were made to rationalize the health care delivery system through a variety of health planning techniques. Prominent among these techniques was the 1975 certificate of need (CON) program that required states to establish systems to limit the expansion of hospital and nursing home facilities and control the diffusion of new technologies.

New systems of care, such as health maintenance organizations (HMOs), were advocated to control costs and serve as a "gatekeeper" to services. Other forms of managed care have evolved during the last twenty years; common to all is the goal of controlling costs by managing service utilization.

Reimbursement for hospital services moved from inflationary cost-based principles to negotiated prospective payment rates. These prospective payment systems as well as state efforts at rate setting to constrain hospital costs for public payors quickly were picked up by private sector payors.

Insurers began to look closely at the services authorized by physicians. Insurance companies invested heavily in cost-saving strategies such as requiring second opinions for surgery, requiring that procedures be approved before admission, and other ways to review procedures and services.

Employers tried to limit their financial exposure by requiring employees to share more costs. Deductibles, copayments, and coinsurance increased patients' out-of-pocket expenses, reversing a thirty-year trend (see Figure 4). Purchasers began to look at managed care to control utilization and payment in an effort to limit their costs. Most important, all payors—public and private—began to shift costs to others and tried to prevent others from shifting costs to them.

WHAT DOES THE SYSTEM LOOK LIKE TODAY?

Today's health care system is a patchwork of multiple public and private financing mechanisms, each with its own rules for eligibility, payment, and coverage. Rather than working cooperatively, the public and private sectors compete, each protecting its own interests and each trying to reduce its own risks and costs. As a result, there are gaps in coverage, duplication of effort, and high administrative costs.

Cost shifting runs rampant. Today there is a hidden tax on those people with insurance, much of which is paid for by employers who

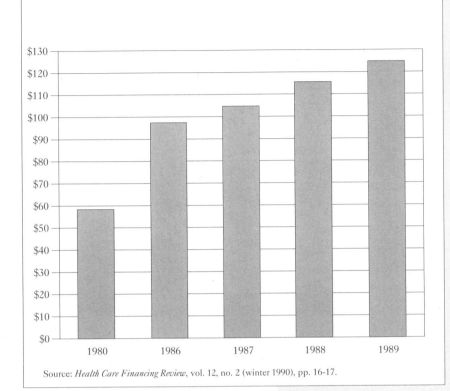

FIGURE 4 OUT-OF-POCKET EXPENSES FOR PERSONAL HEALTH CARE IN THE UNITED STATES, 1980–1989

Source: *Health Care Financing Review*, vol. 12, no. 2 (winter 1990), pp. 16-17.

offer insurance, to pay for the workers of employers not offering insurance and for the coverage and funding gaps in public programs.

The health care reimbursement system is fragmented and provides no real way to contain costs. While one payor or purchaser may reduce its costs in the short term, the lack of a unified reimbursement system leads to further cost shifting. Ultimately there are no real structural incentives for providers to become more efficient.

The employer-based system has made working Americans almost entirely dependent on their employers for coverage. So, whether an individual employee gets insurance depends on the size, nature, and profitability of a business—as well as on the health experience of its employees. This problem is compounded by the fact that small businesses—the fastest growing employers in the country—often are the least able to afford insurance and may have to pay the most for coverage.

Finally, private health insurance has become less of a vehicle for taking risks than for avoiding them. Those most in need of insurance may be either excluded entirely or forced to pay very high, often unaffordable premiums.

The public sector is experiencing similar problems and has responded in much the same way. Concerns about costs have led to limits on the number of people eligible for public programs; to payment mechanisms that limit cross-subsidies to other payors; and to tightened payments to providers, which have led many to stop serving public clients. These responses are reflected in the experience of Medicare and Medicaid during the past twenty-five years. Categorical restrictions in the Medicaid program have kept people out of the system, and reimbursement controls have minimized the costs for those who are in the system. Proposals to expand Medicare to meet the needs of the elderly have been resisted, and recipient cost sharing has been increased while provider payments have been reduced.

The players in the "system" have become so concerned with the issues of financing, coverage, risk aversion, and cost shifting that few have stopped to ask the critical questions for reform:

✦ What kind of services should be accessible to all citizens if the nation is to achieve the vision of health for all by the year 2000?

✦ What kind of service delivery system will best provide those services?

✦ How can the nation equitably finance those services and that delivery system across all sectors of the economy?

✦ Will these efforts result in better health for all Americans?

WHAT CAN GOVERNORS DO?

Governors control a number of policy levers that can be used to improve access, ensure quality, and control costs. These levers give them wide authority and responsibility to allocate human and financial resources in the health care system.

The state role in health care derives from its authority and responsibility to protect the health and welfare of citizens. Historically, state and local governments were the primary actors in publicly funded health programs. It was not until 1965, with the passage of Medicare and Medicaid, that federal spending on health surpassed state and local spending. Although the federal government's role in health care has expanded greatly, states retain most of the authority and responsibility for administering health programs.

Financing and Delivering Services Through Public Health

Long the province of state government, traditional public health encompasses a range of preventive and curative health services aimed at protecting and improving the health and well-being of all Americans. Within this broad scope are efforts to control communicable diseases through immunizations; monitor health and identify the onset of epidemics through the collection of health statistics; screen for infectious diseases such as venereal disease and AIDS; and provide education for prevention and health promotion.

Within each state, the state health department has primary responsibility for ensuring public health. As ensurers and providers of preventive health services, state health agencies play an important role in the total health care system.

Financing and Delivering Services Through Medicaid and Alternative Settings

Paying for care accounts for the greatest proportion of state dollars spent on health activities. While most attention is focused on the size and growth of the Medicaid program, states also devote significant general revenue to special populations. Spending is primarily for programs based on income, age, or specific conditions.

Provisions in state constitutions or statutes make state governments responsible for caring for the indigent. In most states this responsibility is carried out through general assistance programs, in addition to Medicaid. General assistance programs typically pay for medical services—usually hospital care—for low-income people who do not have public or private insurance. Another significant area of state activity is providing health and social services to the frail elderly. Almost every state has programs that pay for services not available through Medicare and Medicaid, and for the elderly not covered by other public or private programs. In addition, states often establish programs designed to meet the needs of people who have a specific medical condition or disease. These include programs for persons with AIDS, Alzheimer's disease, or sickle-cell anemia, and for ventilator-dependent children.

State and local governments also develop direct service delivery systems. Direct delivery takes place through a network of public providers, including hospitals, nursing homes, clinics, and physicians. At the state level the primary sources of this care are state university hospitals and state hospitals providing inpatient mental health, alcohol and drug treatment, and developmental disability services. Increasingly, states are turning to community-based clinics for delivering primary and preventive services.

Regulating Providers

States regulate service providers by setting criteria for state licensure and certification. This authority applies to both professions and facilities. States can also create new kinds of providers such as care coordinators, nurse-midwives, and physician assistants.

States also play a role in educating providers. State universities train physicians, nurses, and other health professionals. A number of states use their educational function to influence where providers deliver services. For example, a number of programs provide scholarship or loan assistance for students who agree to serve in rural areas.

States regulate the allocation of capital investments. Most states have a process for determining the investment in, and allocation of, new technology and new facilities. States can regulate not only cost, but also the location of capital investment. This makes it possible for states to improve the availability of services in underserved areas. States also play a role in restructuring health care facilities. Ambulatory surgical centers, hospices, and rural medical assistance facilities are examples of new types of health care facilities developed in states.

States regulate payment to providers and have developed innovative payment mechanisms that have served as models for the federal government and private purchasers. A number of states have reformed their service payment methods to provide incentives for providers to deliver care in more appropriate and less costly settings. Finally, in addition to payment methods, states have developed innovative case management systems to control costs and monitor the utilization of services.

Regulating Insurance

State government regulates insurance, generally, and health insurance, specifically. The foundation for the state role is the protection of its citizens—in this case, insurance policyholders.

Regulations ensure that insurance companies are financially solvent. State laws and regulations establish standardized definitions of terms of coverage. States also have the authority to ensure that policies do not contain provisions that are unfair, inequitable, deceptive, or misleading. Finally, states determine which benefits must be included in health insurance plans.

A major constraint on state authority, however, results from the federal pension reform law—the Employee Retirement Income Security Act (ERISA). ERISA exempts all self-insured employee health plans from state regulation. Because more than 50 percent of U.S. firms self-insure, states face some limits on their attempts at comprehensive health care reform.

Providing Benefits to State Employees

State government directly insures more than 4 million active employees and retirees. As major employers, states have become caught in the same cost spiral as their private counterparts.

Like private employers, state governments use a variety of cost containment strategies. Most states self-insure their employee benefit plans, as do most large employers. States have moved away from paying total premium costs by requiring employee contributions, especially for family coverage. Finally, there is an increasing trend for states to promote greater HMO participation, and a heightened interest in other managed care arrangements.

HOW CAN THIS REPORT HELP?

The premise of this report is that it will be some years before a national consensus is reached about how best to reform the nation's health care system. It also assumes that no Governor can afford to wait for national consensus before taking action.

The report, therefore, not only raises and explores the significant problems in the health care system, but also provides concrete options that states can employ to:

✦ Focus their health care system to provide systematic and routine preventive and primary care services for all citizens;

✦ Develop ways to both encourage and assist businesses in finding affordable and available health insurance for their employees, and to stabilize coverage for employees already receiving health insurance;

✦ Identify the unique needs of the disparate populations who comprise the nonworking uninsured and develop systems of care to address those needs;

✦ Make better use of incremental cost control strategies that currently are available to every Governor;

✦ Take bold steps to implement major structural changes in the health care system at the state level to significantly check the rise in health care costs; and

✦ Seize the opportunity to move beyond the current system to develop a financing and service delivery system that provides access to all at affordable prices.

State government occupies a crucial position in protecting the health and welfare of Americans. State government is both large enough to develop an effective health system, and small enough to be sensitive to the diverse needs of the people. Therefore, states are the appropriate sites for developing prototypes for health care reform; such state experimentation can lay a solid foundation for the development of national consensus.

The costs of inaction are high. The nation cannot afford to leave the current health care system as it is. And Governors cannot wait for a national consensus before implementing serious reform. Without significant change at the state level, Governors increasingly will be faced with spiraling costs that rob them of the freedom and flexibility to invest in other issues that are vital for a healthy citizenry and a productive economy. If steps are not taken now to build a workable health care system, too many children will continue to come to school unprepared to learn, too many adolescents will continue to face serious but preventable health problems, and too many adults will be prevented from leading full and productive lives.

ENDNOTES

1. Richard Darman, Director, Office of Management and Budget, *Testimony on The Problem of Rising Health Costs*, before the U.S. Senate Finance Committee, April 16, 1991, p. 6.

2. A. Foster Higgins and Co., Inc., *Health Care Benefits Survey 1990* (Princeton, N.J.: A. Foster Higgins and Co., Inc., 1990).

3. U.S. House of Representatives, Committee on Ways and Means, *Overview of Entitlement Programs: 1991 Green Book* (Washington, D.C.: U.S. Government Printing Office, May 7, 1991).

4. Marcia A. Howard, *Fiscal Survey of the States* (Washington, D.C.: National Governors' Association and National Association of State Budget Officers, April 1991).

5. Howard, p. ix.

6. Jill D. Foley, *Uninsured in the United States: The Nonelderly Population without Health Insurance* (Washington, D.C.: Employee Benefit Research Institute, April 1991).

7. "New Worries About Old Diseases," *Newsweek*, May 27, 1991.

8. Paul Starr, *The Social Transformation of American Medicine* (New York: Basic Books, 1982), pp. 198-234, 290-378.

9. Health Insurance Association of America, *Source Book of Health Insurance Data*, 1990 (Washington, D.C.: Health Insurance Association of America, 1990), pp. 23, 40-43.

Focusing on Preventive and Primary Care

SUMMARY   Preventive and primary care services are the base of the health care system. At present, the base is not broad or deep enough to support the massive health care structure built on top of it. The nation cannot continue to invest more and more health care resources in marginally effective services while neglecting services that can have a dramatic effect on the health and productivity of society. Scarce health dollars can be better spent for services such as preventive and primary care that promote and maintain health. This requires not only a change in the philosophical underpinning of the health care system to focus on prevention, but also a reallocation of health resources.

For too many people care is available only when their health condition reaches a crisis level, but not before, when the crisis might have been averted. Access to preventive and primary care health services, as with other health services, is highly inequitable. Yet the burden of disease falls most heavily on those who have the least access to the health care system at the point when appropriate services potentially have the most positive effects. Basic health services should be available and accessible to all Americans, regardless of their age, sex, race, economic status, or geographic location.

WHY ARE PREVENTIVE AND PRIMARY CARE IMPORTANT?

Premature death, illness, and disability exact a heavy toll on the quality of life, economic productivity, and general well-being of individuals, families, and society (see Table 2). This nation has the ability to avert the needless and premature loss of life by using proven strategies for health promotion and disease prevention, and by providing timely primary health services. During the last decade, rates of several of the leading causes of death have declined, reflecting attention to risk factors, such as high blood pressure detection, declines in cigarette smoking, increased use of seat belts, and decreased consumption of fat in the diet. The fact that the death rates have declined should not lessen the demand for preventive and primary care services but further stimulate other activities that can make a difference.

✦ Nearly 57 million persons are injured each year at a cost of $158 billion. The productivity losses from injuries exceed those from heart disease, cancer, and stroke. Most of the injuries occur to the most vulnerable populations—children and the elderly.[1]

✦ Cigarette smoking accounts for more than 434,000 premature deaths and 1.2 million years of potential life lost each year. It is the leading cause of preventable illness and death in the United States.[2]

✦ Sophisticated technology to diagnose and treat disease has outstripped society's ability to pay for it. But many of these expenses would be avoidable if currently available preventive strategies were used to prevent the disease.

◆ It is estimated that infections occurring during hospitalization add $4 billion to national health care costs each year. This affects at least 6 percent of patients admitted to U.S. hospitals and adds at least four days and $1,800 to their hospital stay.[3]

Preventive and primary care are not a panacea for solving the nation's health care crisis, nor are they the only way to improve poor health. Access to health care, even the appropriate level of health care, cannot overcome the negative health consequences of broader social and environmental problems such as poverty, poor housing, and degradation of the environment. Nonetheless, if preventive and primary care services are the foundation of the health care system, they can empower both the individual and the community and thus may pay dividends far beyond the health sector.

Building this foundation necessitates a systemwide philosophical change—a focus on preserving and enhancing the conditions in which people can be healthy. *Healthy People 2000*, a Public Health Service report identifying 298 specific measurable health objectives or targets to be achieved by the year 2000, presents a realistic picture of what the nation can achieve in improved health status through proven interventions.[4] States can be leaders in implementing strategies to achieve these objectives. The benefits of health promotion, protection, and preventive services are promising. No new technologies or methods are required—it is a matter of applying individual and community will together with the resources.

TABLE 2 COSTS OF TREATMENT FOR
SELECTED PREVENTABLE CONDITIONS

Condition	Overall Magnitude	Avoidable Intervention[1]	Cost Per Patient[2]
Heart disease	7 million with coronary artery disease 500,000 deaths per year 284,000 bypass procedures per year	Coronary bypass surgery	$30,000
Cancer	1 million new cases per year	Lung cancer treatment	$29,000
	510,000 deaths per year	Cervical cancer treatment	$28,000
Stroke	600,000 strokes per year 150,000 deaths per year	Hemiplegia treatment and rehabilitation	$22,000
Injuries	2.3 million hospitalizations per year	Quadriplegia treatment and rehabilitation	$570,000 (lifetime)
	142,500 deaths per year	Hip fracture treatment and rehabilitation	$40,000
	177,000 persons with spinal cord injuries in the United States	Severe head injury treatment and rehabilitation	$310,000
HIV infection	1 million–1.5 million infected 118,000 AIDS cases (as of January 1990)	AIDS treatment	$75,000
Alcoholism	18.5 million abuse alcohol 105,000 alcohol-related deaths per year	Liver transplant	$250,000
Drug abuse	Regular users: 1 million–3 million, cocaine 900,000, IV drugs 500,000, heroin Drug-exposed babies: 375,000	Treatment of drug-affected baby	$63,000 (5 years)
Low-birth-weight baby	260,000 low-birthweight babies born per year 23,000 deaths per year	Neonatal intensive care for low-birthweight baby	$10,000
Inadequate	Lacking basic immunization series: 20–30%, age 2 and younger	Congenital rubella syndrome treatment	$354,000 (lifetime)

Notes: [1]Examples (other interventions may apply). [2]Representative first-year costs, except as noted. Not indicated are non-medical costs, such as lost productivity to society.

Source: U.S. Department of Health and Human Services, Public Health Service, *Healthy People 2000* (Washington, D.C.: U.S. Department of Health and Human Services, September 1990).

HEALTHY PEOPLE 2000 GOALS

The U.S. Public Health Service is committed to bringing the nation to its full potential by achieving the following goals:

✦ Increase the span of healthy life for Americans.

✦ Reduce health disparities among Americans.

✦ Achieve access to preventive services for all Americans.

Objectives to meeting these goals fall into the categories of health promotion, which are related to individual lifestyle; health protection, which are those strategies related to environmental or regulatory measures to protect large communities; and preventive services. Specific strategies for meeting these goals include improving indicators in the following areas: maternal and infant health, heart disease and stroke, cancer, diabetes and chronic disabling conditions, HIV infection, sexually transmitted diseases, and immunizations. In addition, the United States must strive to expand access and use of clinical preventive services by eliminating financial barriers.

Traditional public health programs, such as environmental sanitation and communicable disease control, are the core of preventive activities. Recent lapses in the support of these core functions have resulted in new epidemics of measles and other communicable diseases that had been controlled. These illnesses needlessly burden the health care system and the families affected by them because they are completely preventable.

Community prevention systems must be strengthened and expanded to safeguard health and educate citizens about their capacities to maintain their health. These services should be available wherever people are— homes, schools, day care centers, work sites, churches, gyms, and other community organizations.

WHAT ARE PREVENTIVE AND PRIMARY CARE?

Prevention and primary care often are lumped together conceptually, and while related, they clearly are not the same. Prevention encompasses activities that:

✦ Block the initiation of a disease or injury (e.g., immunizations or injury prevention programs);

✦ Alter the impact of a disease after it has begun but before there are recognizable symptoms (e.g., newborn phenylketonuria (PKU) testing identifies infants born with this genetic disorder so that early treatment can prevent mental retardation); and

✦ Limit the disability and suffering associated with chronic illnesses.

Many classic population-based prevention programs have traditionally been conducted by state and local health departments. Such programs include mass immunizations against disease; prevention and control programs for communicable diseases such as AIDS; the assessment of risks to the population posed by various environmental hazards; screening programs such as mammography, hypertension, and blood glucose to enable early identification of symptoms; diagnosis and treatment of chronic diseases; the control of general health threats posed by food-borne or water-borne diseases; the collection and evaluation of health statistics to enable the development of new and better prevention strategies; the development and provision of health education programs aimed at encouraging healthful lifestyles; and the provision of basic preventive services such as prenatal and well-child care to those with no other source of care.

Primary care and prevention overlap to a degree. Certainly many preventive services can and should take place in comprehensive primary care settings. Such settings include federally supported community, migrant, and homeless health centers, rural health centers, local health department clinics, school health clinics, and work site and company clinics.

Primary care services include the evaluation, counseling, health education, diagnostic, and treatment services provided in community settings to prevent, treat, or monitor acute or chronic disease or disability or to prevent premature death. Primary care is continuous and comprehensive and requires collaboration among many health professionals. Primary care physicians include general practitioners, family practitioners, general pediatricians, general internists, and obstetrician-gynecologists. Other primary care providers include licensed nurse-midwives, nurse practitioners, physician assistants, nutritionists, social workers, and health educators.

Comprehensive primary care stresses a gatekeeping function that manages a patient's entire condition rather than just providing a set of services. This gives the patient a health care "home," enabling providers to identify patients' medical, nutritional, emotional, and social needs; treat them; refer some to other appropriate sources of medical and supportive care; and coordinate their care. A comprehensive approach to health is especially important in view of evidence that 30 to 60 percent of visits to primary care physicians are for nonserious medical conditions.[5] While most primary care occurs in physicians' offices, this

definition recognizes that other practitioners can and do provide these services. Finally, although it identifies a constellation of services, the definition is dynamic and undoubtedly will change as more services shift to outpatient settings.

ARE PREVENTIVE AND PRIMARY CARE COST-EFFECTIVE?

While there is compelling evidence that preventive and primary care are cost-effective, need and fairness also should be evaluation criteria. For example, basic childhood health supervision by trained providers can be supported based on concerns about quality and equity, even if it has not yet been proven unequivocally to save long-term costs.

Evidence of the cost-effectiveness of preventive and primary care includes the following.

✦ For every dollar spent on prenatal care, more than three dollars can be saved in the first year of a child's life.[6]

✦ Immunizations can save even greater costs of illness, complications, and death. The measles, mumps, and rubella vaccine is estimated to save fourteen dollars for every dollar spent on immunization.[7] And even with higher costs associated with product liability, the whooping cough vaccine produces a positive benefit-cost ratio.

✦ Work-site treatment and monitoring of high blood pressure has been estimated to save from two to four dollars for every dollar spent.[8]

✦ Programs to help diabetics manage their illness and reduce costly and life-threatening complications have been shown to save more than twice their cost.[9]

✦ Targeted smoking cessation programs, such as those aimed at pregnant women, have proven cost-effective.[10]

There is a need for still more research on the effectiveness and health outcomes of preventive and primary care.

WHAT IS THE STATUS OF PREVENTIVE AND PRIMARY CARE SERVICES?

Despite the importance and effectiveness of preventive and primary care, intrinsic barriers within the health care system often make it hard to provide basic health services. Currently, far more incentives exist within the health care system to provide services at the highest and costliest level than incentives to intervene at an earlier point. This is a critical area states can address by stimulating the effective organization and delivery of preventive and primary care services.

De-emphasis of Community-Based Services

As health care costs have escalated, a relatively smaller portion of health care expenditures have been invested in highly effective communitywide interventions such as school-based immunizations and communicable disease control. The result is a de-emphasis on services that are broadly applicable and very effective. Not only has the relative portion of funds appropriated to community-based services declined, but provision of these services has suffered from changes in society that make communities difficult to define and hard to organize. Community-based services place a premium on communities acting together for the common good.

Disparities in Access to Care

Not all people have access to preventive and primary care services. Differences exist by race, income, economic status, age, insurance status, and geographic location. While these differences do not completely explain the wide disparities in health status among various population groups, they do identify groups to whom services could be targeted.

✦ In 1986 almost one-quarter (24 percent) of pregnant women had not begun prenatal care in the first trimester. While almost 80 percent of white women received early care, only 61 percent of black and Hispanic women started prenatal care early. The uninsured and those in public programs (primarily Medicaid) were more likely than the privately insured to have late prenatal care or none at all.[11]

✦ While the use of preventive care by poor black women has been increasing, other poor and uninsured women are considerably less likely than higher income or insured women to have a blood pressure reading, a Pap smear, or breast examination by a physician.[12] A recent study found that 66 percent of women between the ages of seventeen to forty-four, and 57 percent of women between the ages of forty-five and sixty-five, received a Pap smear at least once in three years, well below the Surgeon General's goal of 85 percent.[13]

✦ Uninsured Americans visit physicians less often than those with health insurance: While 75 percent of insured Americans had at least one doctor visit in 1984, only 60 percent of the uninsured saw a doctor.[14] Even when adjusted for health status, the uninsured are less likely to receive physician care, and the elderly without insurance that supplements Medicare also are less likely to visit a physician.[15] The uninsured who are poor are considerably less likely to receive physician services.[16] Poor blacks and Hispanics are somewhat less likely to have a physician visit, despite worse health status.[17]

✦ For the 20 percent of the population residing in rural areas, problems of access have been exacerbated by the closure of hundreds of rural health care facilities in recent years.

Limited Physician Attention to Preventive Care

Private physicians traditionally have not emphasized health promotion—counseling patients in healthy behavior and risk reduction—beyond physical check-ups. Few physicians refer patients to preventive care providers or employ clinical staff, such as nurses, who provide it. Physicians are trained to solve existing problems, not anticipate and avoid future ones. Limited reimbursement, lack of training, conflicting evidence on the efficacy of some services, lack of confidence in their ability to change patient behavior, the belief that patients do not want to hear the message, and a lack of time all discourage physicians from focusing on prevention.

Reluctance of Some Public Health Agencies to Deliver Primary Care

Some in the public health community resist an expanded primary care role. They believe that providing primary and acute care for the poor and underserved deprives other vital public health functions—such as health surveillance, control of epidemics, and environmental monitoring—of political and financial capital. Others argue that delivering primary care is not their primary function and choose a more limited role of providing traditional preventive care (immunizations, prena-

143,227

tal care, and well-child or well-adult care). Deciding whether to provide primary care services in public health units is controversial and involves philosophical differences regarding resource allocation.

Public health agencies always have to scrape for resources for community prevention activities because these efforts are invisible to the public. If they take on indigent care services, this may distort their public image and inhibit their ability to maintain community prevention functions. Some public health departments believe the benefits to be gleaned from an expanded role outweigh these concerns.

Emergency Rooms as a Regular Source of Care

People use hospital emergency rooms for nonemergency and emergency care because these facilities have convenient hours of operation and are located near transportation routes, and because they lack other providers. Emergency department use has increased since the 1960s, but most care sought there is not for true emergencies.

Emergency rooms are not the appropriate site for primary and preventive care. They generally do not provide preventive services, are very costly, and do not offer continuity of care.

Shortage of Primary Care Providers

Despite an expected overall surplus of physicians, the proportion of physicians practicing primary care has declined since 1960. Some primary care specialties actually will face shortages in the next decade. The American Medical Association predicts that patient demand will exceed supply for general and family practitioners. In many areas around the country these shortages are critical.

Rural Areas. Recruiting and retaining rural providers present multiple challenges:

✦ Lower expected income due to a smaller population base and poorer patients;

✦ Inadequate income to pay overhead and liability insurance, and repay medical loans.

✦ A lack of training and preparation for rural practice;

✦ Limited availability of nearby hospitals or hospitals with advanced technology;

✦ Professional isolation (i.e., few colleagues with whom to share responsibilities and expertise); and

✦ A lack of amenities for providers and their families compared with metropolitan areas.

Health care services often are not integrated in rural communities, so patients have to leave home to seek care from distant hospitals and outpatient providers. Although mid-level practitioners could provide preventive and primary care in rural areas, their scope of practice is restricted. Physician supervision standards and limited prescribing privileges in many states impede wider use of physician assistants and nurse practitioners. Moreover, continuing education requirements for mid-level practitioners are more difficult to fulfill in rural areas.

Urban Areas. Rural communities are not the nation's only underserved areas. Big cities also face shortages of physicians, while nearby suburbs are oversupplied. From 1963 to 1980, the number of office-based primary care physicians in urban poverty areas declined, while the number of hospital-based physicians increased somewhat.[18] Although distances are not as great as in rural areas, limited public transportation makes it hard for inner-city residents to reach suburban physi-cian offices. Instead, they turn to more accessible hospital emergency departments. Physicians are less likely to set up inner-city practices due to limited earnings potential and cultural and language differences that may impede communication with and treatment of patients. Minority physicians are more likely to establish practices in underserved urban areas, and thus the decline in the number of minority medical students is troubling because it may compound physician shortages in these locations.

Physician Reluctance to Participate in Public Programs

Even communities served by adequate numbers of primary care physicians face shortages of doctors willing to serve patients under public programs. While pediatricians have been among the most willing Medicaid providers, a 1990 survey showed that their participation declined from 85 percent in 1978 to 77 percent in 1989.[19] Recent federal mandates to raise fees for obstetrical and pediatric services may stem further losses, but may not entice dissatisfied physicians back into the program.

Malpractice and Access to Care

One of the most disturbing consequences of rising malpractice costs has been the impact on access to care, particularly for low-income individuals. The rising cost of malpractice insurance has reportedly led many physicians to avoid high-risk patients and refuse to perform certain procedures. Many physicians are changing specialties, contributing to a shortage of providers in vital primary care specialties, such as family practice and obstetrics. The shortage of obstetricians is an area of particular concern given the increased emphasis states have been placing on prenatal care.

The Cost of Care

While many nonfinancial barriers deter access to needed preventive and primary care, cost remains the major barrier. A national study of blood pressure screening, Pap smears, clinical breast examination, and glaucoma tests among middle-aged women concluded that insurance coverage was the single most important predictor of whether someone uses preventive care. Lack of insurance coverage reduced the chance that women would use these services by about 50 percent.[20]

Cost is a major barrier for poor children who need preventive and primary care and prescribed drugs. When adjusted for their poorer health status, lower income children have considerably fewer physician visits than children from higher income families, and black children have fewer visits than white children do.[21] Despite its limitations, Medicaid coverage improves access to physician care for poor children.

Inadequate Financing Through Insurance

Preventive and primary care services still are not recognized by most reimbursement schemes in the United States. Failure to cover such services is the result of several factors.

✦ Some dispute the value of preventive care.

✦ Many in the insurance industry question whether preventive care is an insurable service since insurance traditionally is designed to protect against major medical outlays due to an unexpected event. Preventive services are neither unpredictable nor, for the most part, extremely costly.

✦ There is some concern that covering these services could lead to abuse by physicians and patients.

Any change in payment systems for preventive care must balance the desire to encourage patients and physicians to use preventive care services appropriately, while avoiding incentives for excessive use or abuse.

The recent measles epidemic highlights the inadequacies of the financing system for preventive services. Even children who have private insurance coverage now are being referred to overburdened public clinics for vaccinations because their insurance does not cover routine immunizations. This has resulted in a decline in the percentage of children fully immunized against childhood diseases and, thus, an increase in preventable diseases such as measles.

WHAT CAN STATES DO TO ENHANCE ACCESS TO PREVENTIVE AND PRIMARY CARE?

States are critical actors in stimulating the transition from a crisis-oriented system to one that focuses on prevention and primary care. Both as investors in the system and innovators within the system, states can make responsible and bold changes in the way health services are organized, delivered, and financed. This will require a reallocation of public and private sector resources to achieve the objectives of *Healthy People 2000*. Even with increased financial coverage through public or private insurance programs, direct public support will be needed for certain elements of the nation's preventive and primary health care delivery system.

State government must ensure that an adequate public health care system exists in every locality. Some communities may never be able to sustain a fully functioning public

COORDINATING CARE IN SOUTH CAROLINA

South Carolina is improving the health of mothers and children through a comprehensive initiative that aggressively reaches out to its consumers. Healthy Mothers–Healthy Futures provides a range of medical and support services to pregnant women and children who are eligible for Medicaid. The major goals of the initiative are to:

✦ Increase primary care physicians' participation in the Medicaid program;

✦ Enhance access to early prenatal care for eligible pregnant women and access to health care for eligible children;

✦ Promote health education during pregnancy; and

✦ Promote referrals to community support programs.

(continued next page)

health department or physician or mid-level practitioner without public subsidies. Some publicly insured patients may have difficulty finding physicians to treat them. And some at-risk populations, such as low-income pregnant women, substance abusers, and the homeless, are better served through a delivery system that addresses more than just medical conditions. In addition to direct public funds for selected health care providers, state government can encourage the use of alternative providers and delivery settings and exert influence over the training, licensing, and placement of health professionals. Training of physicians could be facilitated by more effective use of federal funds, such as Title VII of the Public Health Service Act and direct medical education adjustments to Medicare payment methods, to complement state health personnel priorities in preventive and primary care.

Foster Community-Based Preventive and Primary Care Services

Community-based preventive and primary care services are those that are available where people are—where they live, work, and play. The closer such services are to people, the more likely they are to be used and the more likely they will have a positive impact.

With their unique focus on the broad forces affecting community health, public health agencies can be the catalyst for local efforts to develop strategies for community-based primary care. Or these agencies can take the lead to coordinate existing fragmented services.

Community health centers are important community-based providers of services. Funded under Section 330 of the Public Health Services Act, these centers provide basic primary medical services in rural and urban areas, including ancillary, preventive, and dental services, to persons with financial, geographic, or cultural barriers to care. Community health centers have a mission to serve the poor in medically underserved areas. These centers have several guiding principles: Their geographic location should be accessible, and transportation should be available to the clinic site; financial barriers to health care should be eliminated or minimized; they should be sensitive to clients' culture and seek user acceptance; and they should have convenient hours. Centers should provide primary care and a full range of health and other human services, either on site or through coordinated referrals.

Similar in mission and scope are migrant health centers, which are funded under Section 329 of the Public Health Services Act. These centers provide comprehensive primary health services to migrant and seasonal farm workers and their dependents. They are linked with hospital and other area health and social services. Health Care for the Homeless programs, funded under Section 340 of the Public Health Services Act, provide emergency and other health services in a setting accessible to homeless persons and are linked to hospitals, mental health services, and social services.

Although community and migrant health centers receive more than 40 percent of their funding from federal grants, states have a great deal of influence. State and local grants provide an average of 10 percent of community and migrant health centers' budgets. Moreover, about 30 percent of all low-income individuals served at community and migrant health centers are Medicaid beneficiaries, and about 20 percent of these centers' revenues come from Medicaid.[22]

The relationships between community and migrant health centers and local health departments can be strengthened so that primary care services can be optimally delivered. Linkages that have been successful include those where clinics share space and are jointly administered and operated. This provides greater opportunities for appropriate referrals between agencies and facilitates the integration of client services.

Many states have recognized the need to develop a health care infrastructure to serve low-income, underserved, or otherwise disadvantaged populations. Several states, such as Colorado, Connecticut, Hawaii, Maine, Massachusetts, and Washington, have appropriated funds directly to community health centers—both federally funded and nonprofit —that have a broad community focus. Public and quasi-public comprehensive clinics can provide appropriate and cost-effective preventive and primary care that reduce hospitalization and emergency room use.

Several states facing the closure of small rural hospitals have helped communities explore alternative uses for these facilities. Montana and several other states have changed licensing laws to permit facilities to limit inpatient care and provide more emergency and triage services, often using mid-level practitioners. Closed hospitals in Colorado and Kansas were reopened as community clinics and family practice residency training sites. Some eastern Washington communities are evaluating their health care needs and restructuring their services to develop more locally relevant services and enable residents to get needed care in the community.

Expand the Role of Local Public Health Agencies

Local public health agencies, which exist in almost all states, could be expanded to provide more preventive and primary care. These agencies perform a wide variety of functions. In some communities, public health departments provide preventive care, such as immunizations, for all residents regardless of income. In others they provide preventive services and prenatal and/or well-child care for low-income families. In some areas, especially in large cities and in southern states, local health departments provide a substantial amount of primary care for underserved populations—the poor, the uninsured, and minorities.

Some public health agencies use large public hospitals to provide comprehensive services. For example, the health department in Dade County, Florida, has developed a consortium that includes the county hospital, county-funded clinics, and independent federally funded community health centers. Through an automated registration database, the network operates a triage system to refer uninsured and low-income patients to appropriate care at the appropriate level. Milwaukee County, Wisconsin, operates a managed care system for general assistance medical clients using the county hospital and two private hospitals. Emergency room and outpatient department staffs refer clients to a county primary care clinic or to hospitalization and specialty care, when needed.

Other counties that do not own hospitals have created comprehensive delivery systems that emphasize preventive and primary care. For example, Palm Beach County, Florida, contracts with community health centers and

(continued from previous page)

Home visiting is a key component of the program. Within fourteen days of discharge from the hospital, all eligible mothers and infants receive a home visit by a physician or nurse to assess environmental, social, and medical needs. During the visit, infant care is discussed, and the nurse or physician ensures that the mother has a postpartum appointment, that the infant has a two-week EPSDT visit, and that referrals to other needed services are made.

Home visits also are made when a pregnant woman misses a prenatal care appointment. Additionally, the state provides a pre-discharge visit to the home of an infant admitted to a neonatal intensive care unit to ensure a safe home environment.

private hospitals for the care of its medically indigent population. Nurses function as case managers to coordinate inpatient and outpatient care. In 1982 Sacramento County, California, became responsible for indigent care previously funded by the state. It expanded the primary care capacity of its health department clinics to treat clients, using nurse case managers to refer cases to contracting hospitals and other providers.

Expand the Use of Schools in the Health Care System

As the one location where children convene regularly, schools are in a unique position to identify children's emotional, social, and physical needs and refer them to appropriate programs. At the very least, schools can serve as a link between children and health services. They also can be a focus for financing family health care, as in new demonstrations in Arkansas and Florida.

In some communities, schools can be the locus of direct health care delivery. School health clinics appear to detect a significant amount of untreated illness, can resolve most needs on site, and can increase immunization rates. Some studies also show that these clinics may be associated with less absenteeism due to illness and with reduced use of alcohol and tobacco.[23]

School health clinics can serve lower income and minority children who are less likely to have a regular source of care. They also perform a particularly useful function in reaching adolescents who traditionally are isolated from the health care system and for whom preventive counseling on risky behaviors is especially important. Although not a model that can work everywhere, these clin-

ics seem to be well accepted in their communities, and their numbers are growing. Schools need not be the actual providers of these case management or clinical services, a function that can often be served by other agencies, but they can provide the site. While some states have limited authority over local schools, they can encourage community discussion of this option.

Increase Physicians' Attention to Preventive Care

Because physician training emphasizes curative medicine, most physician practice focuses on therapy rather than prevention. Physicians often are uncomfortable counseling patients about lifestyle and risky behavior, yet such discussions can improve health status. For example, as part of a study of insurance payment for clinical preventive care, physicians participated in educational seminars and received instruction about appropriate preventive care services. Patients in the study used more preventive services and experienced significantly reduced risk factors related to smoking, exercise, seat belts, and breast self-examinations than a control group who were not counseled.[24]

To improve physician participation in clinical preventive services, states can promote professional educational activities, continuing education that includes clinical prevention protocols, medical school curriculum changes, more third-party financing of preventive care, and private sector funding of education and training programs in preventive medicine. States also can encourage the medical profession to collaborate in public relations activities with nonprofit and other organizations to foster prevention, behavioral change, and appropriate use of medical care.

Expand the Supply of Primary Care Practitioners

States with a shortage of various types of preventive and primary care providers in given communities have several options to expand personnel supply.

Train More Primary Care Physicians. Medical students choose specialties other than primary care due to financial concerns and their hospital-based training experience. States can encourage medical students to enter primary care through targeted loan forgiveness and scholarship programs. More opportunities for medical students to experience primary care in office settings can expose them to the challenges and attraction of primary care practice. Although most states now support family practice residency training programs, more widespread use of such programs could offer practical training in real clinical situations. Collaboration with community health centers and other primary care clinics can supplement the physician services in these settings, while acquainting residents with the needs of lower income patients.

Improve Health Personnel Distribution in Rural Areas. A recent Office of Technology Assessment (OTA) report on rural health care suggests that because rural areas experience a variety of problems, different policies may be required to address temporary rather than long-term personnel shortages and varying needs for medical education, technical assistance, and financial support.[25] OTA's report specifically underscores a role for states in identifying areas of need and "enabling states and localities to adopt and adapt programs tailored to their own needs." States also can recruit rural residents into medical and nursing schools and use residency training rotations in rural communities to familiarize young physicians with rural health care needs as well as provide primary care to underserved communities. Medical school training could include specific rotations through rural practice sites. In addition, medical school faculty could rotate through rural and other underserved areas to provide needed peer interaction for practitioners in underserved areas.

Loan and Scholarship Programs. Nineteen states have developed programs to encourage rural primary care practice that are similar to the National Health Service Corps. Most will pay back or forgive student loans if physicians, and sometimes nurses, practice for a given period in rural underserved communities. A few states offer scholarships conditioned on rural service. Indiana and South Dakota provide direct grants to encourage rural practice. North Carolina and Tennessee help rural family practitioners and obstetricians pay malpractice insurance premiums. Under 1990 amendments to the Public Health Service Act, federal funds are available to match state funds for loan repayment, providing an opportunity for more states to address shortages of primary health care personnel in rural and other underserved communities.

Since state programs are new, evidence of their effectiveness is limited. However, Nevada and Wisconsin report very high retention rates for physicians, nurses, and mid-level practitioners. It is important to evaluate these state initiatives to determine which strategies work best and whether states will still need to assume long-term responsibility for grants and scholarships to retain providers in rural areas.

ENHANCED PRENATAL CARE IN DELAWARE

Delaware is one of thirty-six states now offering enhanced prenatal care services through Medicaid. The Smart Start program provides care coordination, risk assessment, nutritional counseling, health education, psychosocial counseling, and home visiting to women at risk of poor pregnancy outcomes.

An initial evaluation of the program found that more than 78 percent of the participating women gave birth to full-term babies, only 14 percent gave birth to low-birthweight babies, and only 3 percent of the babies were born with congenital anomalies. These data suggest that the right interventions delivered at the appropriate time can go a long way toward preventing bad birth outcomes and infant mortality.

Other Incentives. States could consider income tax credits to encourage health care providers to practice in underserved areas. Oregon recently enacted such a credit for rural physicians, nurses, and physician assistants who meet prescribed criteria. States also can provide supplemental payments under Medicaid or other indigent care programs to reward rural practice. This approach could be structured similar to one under Medicare, which pays physicians in health manpower shortage areas a 10 percent bonus above regular fees. The effectiveness of this incentive to encourage rural practice, however, has not been evaluated. Many states also provide recruitment and placement services that help communities locate and attract physicians.

Expand the Use of Mid-Level Practitioners. Physician assistants and nurse practitioners have tended to locate disproportionately in small rural communities. Furthermore, there is evidence that these practitioners are more likely to stay in rural communities and that they provide high-quality care, excelling in services involving patient communication. Expanding their capability to practice in underserved areas, particularly rural areas, could meet some of the need for preventive and primary care providers.

In 1990 Kentucky authorized the development of licensed health care networks based in clinics or physicians' offices and linked to other medical and related community services. These networks are expected to rely heavily on the services of mid-level practitioners at local sites who will work under the indirect supervision of a primary care physician.

Virginia recently enacted a law allowing nurse-midwives to prescribe certain drugs. Although allowing these practitioners to prescribe these drugs makes them more able to provide full-service prenatal care, fewer than half the states authorize such prescribing. While there may be some resistance from physicians, where primary care shortages are significant, states can review licensing laws to expand the scope of practice by mid-level providers or reduce requirements for physician supervision. Increasing access should not sacrifice quality of care. States also can encourage the use of mid-level providers through direct reimbursement for their services under Medicaid in settings other than certified rural health clinics. This has been done in some states. Moreover, all states are required to directly reimburse nurse practitioners participating in Medicaid.

Decrease Malpractice Insurance Costs

Several states have provided malpractice subsidies to obstetricians in an effort to promote care in underserved areas. Some states have created no-fault funds for certain classes of obstetric care. Others also have protected obstetricians who serve low-income populations under "good Samaritan" laws that exempt these physicians from liability. Missouri allows some primary care physicians practicing in public programs to receive liability coverage under the state legal expense fund, thus removing physicians' public service population from their private liability.

Mandate Preventive and Primary Care in Private Insurance Plans

Private insurers have begun to cover selected preventive services, but such coverage still is not the norm. States can expand preventive care insurance benefits by adopting insurance mandates or other incentives. Such mandates should be considered only based on a set of explicit criteria (e.g., cost-effectiveness). A few states mandate that group (and often individual) insurance cover services such as mammography (thirteen states), well-child care (six states), Pap smears (five states), and diabetes education (six states).[26]

Opponents of insurance mandates are concerned that these requirements raise insurance costs and encourage employers to self-insure. Self-insured employers are beyond the reach of state regulation. They argue that mandates in general result in extra spending due to the phenomenon of "moral hazard," the tendency for an insured person to consume more services (e.g., medical care) because insurance lowers the marginal cost of services. However, some services, such as mammography, save long-term health care costs, which weakens these arguments.

Despite the limited evidence on the costs and benefits of other preventive care services, states might want to establish protocols for the frequency of services and require that all insured children be covered for at least a minimum number of preventive visits. States considering this option might want to package appropriate preventive services into a single insurance requirement rather than perpetuate the piecemeal enactment of individual mandates. If protocols are developed for other populations, determinations about what are appropriate preventive services could be related to age. For example, women past their child-bearing years will not need prenatal care, but will need coverage for mammographies.

Incentives to encourage alternative insurance that still offers desirable benefits are found in laws permitting insurers to sell small employer policies that are exempt from most state insurance mandates (e.g., care for mental health and substance abuse). Of the ten states that authorize such bare-bones small group insurance plans, Oklahoma specifically requires policies to include prenatal care, and Virginia requires maternity and well-child care, services not otherwise required. States considering such limited coverage authority can tie it to small group health insurance market reform and can condition benefit limits on the expansion of selected preventive services that further policy objectives, such as increasing access to basic care for women and children.

Improve Early and Periodic Screening, Diagnostic, and Treatment Services

The Health Care Financing Administration's new EPSDT participation goals require most states to re-examine their program administration. A recent National Governors' Association report on prospects for improving EPSDT's mission found that newly eligible children often are not enrolled in Medicaid, and even when enrolled, do not use the EPSDT benefit for several reasons:

✦ Medicaid's complex application process;

✦ Families' lack of understanding of the importance of preventive care; and

✦ The focus of outreach efforts on pregnant women, rather than children.

ACCESS TO
OBSTETRICAL CARE IN
WEST VIRGINIA

*With support from the Robert
Wood Johnson Foundation,
West Virginia has begun a
program to provide financial
assistance to nurses interested
in furthering their education
to become certified midwives.
The state also is pursuing
the establishment of a School of
Midwifery at the Marshall
Medical School of the University
of West Virginia. By the end
of 1992, more certified nurse-
midwives than family
practitioners will be practicing
in the state. Access to obstetrical
care, especially for indigent
women, will be greatly
improved.*

State outreach and eligibility simplification activities to enroll eligible low-income pregnant women now are serving as a model to increase public awareness of the value of preventive care for children and the availability of Medicaid to finance care. The NGA report cites numerous examples of state strategies to improve children's enrollment in Medicaid and overcome the deterrent effects of complex application forms and procedures: placing eligibility workers at provider sites; shortening application forms; waiving assets tests; expediting application processing; permitting applications to be mailed; using care coordinators; initiating statewide preventive and primary care outreach campaigns; and coordinating eligibility under related public programs. The report also notes the need for improvements in ensuring that children with identified conditions are referred for treatment and for collaboration with other maternal and child health agencies, especially those serving chronically ill children.

Improve Physician Medicaid Participation

Past reports of the National Governors' Association have examined options for states to improve physician participation in Medicaid, especially obstetricians.[27] Some states have changed the tort recovery system or provided other ways to lower medical malpractice premiums for physicians treating public patients. The recent report on children identifies state efforts to attract and retain pediatric providers. These strategies are similar to those states have used to attract and retain obstetrical providers. For example, some states are increasing pediatric service fees, and many are streamlining billing procedures or establishing electronic billing systems to respond to physi-

cian concerns about paperwork, payment delays, and reimbursement levels. Because Medicaid eligibility is ineffectual without provider participation, these issues require continuing state attention.

Encourage Private Philanthropy

Private philanthropy supported a small fraction of personal health care in 1988, mostly hospital care, though many community clinics and nonprofit nursing agencies are very substantially supported by philanthropic contributions. To encourage more preventive and primary care for children, Blue Cross Associations in twelve states match privately raised funds to finance ambulatory care for uninsured low-income children provided through Blue Cross's physician networks. Although most of these programs, called Caring Foundations, operate independently of state government, Michigan's program is collaborating with Medicaid to fund children's health care, and Iowa appropriated seed money to get Blue Cross's project started there. Colorado is funding a new children's health plan by matching public with private funds. Even without financial support, public officials in other states can encourage these types of private sector efforts.

Set an Example

States can set an example by emphasizing preventive and primary care services in tangible ways. For example, states can:

✦ Require seat belt use by state employees;

✦ Make state offices smoke-free environments; and

✦ Operate effective employee assistance programs for state employees.

After Preventive and Primary Care Services, What Next?

States have many options to increase the availability and accessibility of preventive and primary care services. Yet access to these and all other services is a function of the strength and breadth of the state's health delivery system, and of one's health insurance status. Health insurance coverage and access to health care are fundamentally linked in the United States. Whether coverage is through the employer-based system or through public programs such as Medicaid, the immediate key to increasing access to care is to identify the gaps in the insurance system—either public or private—that exclude many people from coverage. The next step is to focus on ways to fill the gaps and overcome some of the practices that exacerbate them.

Endnotes

1. Dorothy P. Rice and Alan J. MacKenzie and Associates, "Cost of Injury in the United States: A Report to Congress, 1989," *Morbidity and Mortality Weekly Reports*, vol. 38, no. 4 (November 3, 1989), pp. 743-746.

2. Centers for Disease Control, "Smoking Attributable Mortality and Years of Potential Life Lost, U.S., 1988," *Mortality and Morbidity Weekly Report*, vol. 40, no. 62.

3. Robert W. Haley, *Managing Hospital Control for Cost-Effectiveness* (Chicago, Ill.: American Hospital Publishing, Inc., 1986).

4. U.S. Department of Health and Human Services, Public Health Service, *Healthy People 2000* (Washington, D.C.: U.S. Department of Health and Human Services, 1990).

5. A.J. Barsky, "The Paradox of Health," *New England Journal of Medicine*, vol. 318, no. 7 (1988), pp. 414-418.

6. Institute of Medicine, *Preventing Low Birthweight* (Washington, D.C.: National Academy Press, 1985); and J. Hadley, E.P. Steinberg, and J. Feder, "Comparison of Uninsured and Privately Insured Hospital Patients," *Journal of the American Medical Association*, vol. 265, no. 3 (1991), pp. 374-379.

7. C.C. White, J.P. Koplan, W.A. Orenstein, "Benefits, Risks, and Costs of Immunizations for Measles, Mumps, and Rubella," *American Journal of Public Health*, vol. 75, no. 7 (1985), pp. 739-744.

8. M. Kristein, "The Economics of Health Promotion at the Worksite," *Health Education Quarterly*, vol. 9 (supplement, 1982), pp. 27-36.

9. Mine Diabetes Control Project, "Impact of Diabetes Outpatient Education Program," *Morbidity and Mortality Weekly Report*, vol. 31, no. 23 (1982), pp. 307-314; T.M. Smeeding, *Measuring and Valuing the Economic Benefits of Diabetes Control: The Economic Perspective* (Salt Lake City, Utah: University of Utah, Department of Economics, April 1983).

10. A. Elixhauser, "The Costs of Smoking and the Cost-Effectiveness of Smoking Cessation Programs," *Journal of Public Health Policy*, summer 1980, pp. 218-237.

11. D. Hughes et al., "The Health of American Children," (Washington, D.C.: Children's Defense Fund, 1989).

12. E.B. Keeler et al., "How Free Care Reduced Hypertension in the Health Insurance Experiment," *Journal of the American Medical Association*, vol. 254, no. 14 (1985), pp. 1926-1931.

13. Davis et al., "Paying for Preventive Care: Moving the Debate Forward," *American Journal of Preventive Medicine*, vol. 6, no. 4 (1990). 14. R. Andersen, M. Chen, L. Aday, L. Cornelius, "Health Status and Medical Care Utilization," *Health Affairs*, vol. 6, no. 1 (1987), pp. 136-156.

15. R. M. Andersen et al., *Ambulatory Care and Insurance Coverage in an Era of Constraint* (Chicago, Ill.: Pluribus Press, 1987).

16. G. Wilensky, "Health Care, the Poor, and the Role of Medicaid," *Health Affairs*, vol. 1, no. 4 (1982), pp. 93-100.

17. G. Hendershot, "Health Status and Medical Care Utilization," *Health Affairs*, vol. 7, no. 1 (1988), pp. 114-121.

18. D.A. Kindig et al., "Trends in Physician Availability in 10 Urban Areas from 1963 to 1980," *Inquiry*, vol. 24, no. 2 (1987), pp. 136-146.

19. Ian Hill and Janine Breyel, *Caring for Kids* (Washington, D.C.: National Governors' Association, 1991).

20. S. Woolhandler and D.U. Himmelstein, "Reverse Targeting of Preventive Care Due to Lack of Health Insurance," *Journal of the American Medical Association*, vol. 259 (1988), pp. 2872-2874.

21. P.W. Newacheck and B. Starfield, "Morbidity and Use of Ambulatory Care Services among Poor Children," *American Journal of Public Health*, vol. 78, no. 8 (1988), pp. 927-933.

22. D. Lewis-Idema, *Factors Influencing Medicaid Reimbursement to Community and Migrant Health Centers* (Washington, D.C.: National Association of Community Health, 1990).

23. Center for Population Options, *School-Based Clinics Enter the '90s: Update, Evaluation, and Future Challenges* (Washington, D.C.: Center for Population Options, 1990).

24. Davis et al., "Paying for Preventive Care: Moving the Debate Forward," *American Journal of Preventive Medicine*, vol. 6, no. 4 (1990).

25. U.S. Congress, Office of Technology Assessment, *Health Care in Rural America* (Washington, D.C.: Office of Technology Assessment, September 1990).

26. Davis et al., "Paying for Preventive Care: Moving the Debate Forward," *American Journal of Preventive Medicine*, vol. 6, no. 4 (1990).

27. Deborah Lewis-Idema, *Increasing Provider Participation* (Washington, D.C.: National Governors' Association, 1988).

Improving EPSDT in Utah

Utah has run a multifaceted perinatal outreach campaign since 1988. Through television and radio announcements, printed material, coupon book, and hotline, the Baby Your Baby campaign has now achieved a 90 percent name recognition rate among Utah residents. Capitalizing on this success, state officials recently launched a second phase of Baby Your Baby, expanding its message to persuade families to obtain early and continuous well-child care.

Following a strategy similar to that used in the first phase, a broad-based coalition of interested groups was formed, including the Utah Department of Health, the local NBC affiliate (KUTV), and an association of independent nonprofit hospitals. Members designed a diverse campaign that incorporates television and radio public service announcements, print advertisements, direct mailings, ongoing correspondence, and patient incentives to communicate the message.

Facilitating the Private Commitment

SUMMARY Most Americans obtain health insurance for themselves and their families through their jobs. Yet 19 million adult workers have no insurance. Since health insurance is a major component of employee compensation, why are so many workers uninsured? In part, it is due to structural changes occurring in the U.S. economy, including the substantial employment growth in service industries, the increase in part-time employment, and the rising number of small businesses. Other factors, such as the escalating cost of insurance, also play a role.

These developments have prompted calls for changes to the current employer-based system to ensure coverage for the working uninsured. States can pursue four approaches to assist these workers in obtaining health insurance:

✦ Require Employers to Offer Health Insurance.

✦ Reduce the Cost of Insurance.

✦ Directly Finance the Cost of Care.

✦ Ensure That the Insurance Market Functions Effectively.

Facilitating coverage for the working uninsured will require a redefinition of the traditional roles played by the private and public sectors. It also will require greater regulation of the market, so it can work freely.

WHO ARE THE WORKING UNINSURED?

Of the estimated 34.4 million nonelderly Americans without health insurance, more than 80 percent are either workers or their dependents.[1] The majority of the working uninsured are employed in small firms that do not offer coverage. For those who are self-employed, the costs of insurance may be prohibitive. Others are per-day, part-time, or seasonal workers who are not eligible for benefits like insurance. Still others have pre-existing conditions or are deemed high-risk, making them uninsurable.

The 19 million adult workers without any employer-group health insurance are predominantly young, earn relatively low weekly wages (in part because they are young workers), typically work all year, and work mostly in service industries. More than 80 percent are between eighteen and forty-four years of age. Roughly half the workers without any employer-group coverage work all year, though 85 percent have weekly earnings below $400, which is less than $20,000 per year.[2] Finally, the service and retail trade industries employ the largest percentages of these workers—for example, in libraries, museums, day care centers, department stores, supermarkets, and restaurants.[3]

Most U.S. workers obtain coverage through their jobs. Health insurance is a major facet of employee compensation and is offered, nearly universally, to full-time employees in medium-sized and large private businesses and state and local governments.[4] However, something appears to have gone awry with the basic premise of this system—that health care coverage is tied to employment. For despite the breadth of employer-based insurance, a significant number of working people and their families do not have protection.

Unfortunately, the situation is not likely to improve on its own. Forces shaping the U.S. economy are continuing to cause changes in the location, hours, and structure of work.[5] These changes, coupled with the ways employers and private insurers are responding to them, have made the problem of the working uninsured more pervasive. Indeed, it is these developments that have led many to call for modifications to the current employer-based health insurance system to ensure coverage for this population.

THE WORKING UNINSURED

✦ *60 percent are men.*

✦ *35 percent are between age 30 and 44.*

✦ *62 percent work a full year with no unemployment.*

✦ *44 percent work in the service and retail industries.*

✦ *50 percent work in firms with fewer than 25 employees or are self-employed.*

✦ *85 percent earn less than $20,000 per year, or $384 a week.*

✦ *86 percent of uninsured children live in homes where the family head works.*

Source: Jill D. Foley, *Uninsured in the United States: The Nonelderly Population without Health Insurance* (Washington, D.C.: Employee Benefit Research Institute, April 1991), pp. 43, 45-46, 49, 54, 67.

WHY HAS THE PROBLEM BECOME SO PERVASIVE?

Ironically, despite the dramatic economic recovery this nation experienced during the last decade, the number of uninsured actually increased. While the economy was expanding, it was also undergoing radical changes.

The Shift to a Service Economy

The U.S. economy has moved from what was largely a manufacturing economy to one that relies more heavily on so-called service industries. The substantial employment growth that has occurred in, for example, wholesale and retail trade and health care and business services, is likely to continue in the foreseeable future. Some of these industries are among those whose workers are the least likely to get coverage through their jobs. In 1990 about 16 million of the working uninsured held nonmanufacturing jobs, compared with about 2 million who were employed in manufacturing industries.[6]

The Rising Number of Small Businesses

The typical service establishment employs only eleven people, compared with the average manufacturing company, which has sixty workers. Since employment gains will be in service industries, most new jobs will be created by small businesses.[7] Of the 10.5 million net new jobs created between 1980 and 1986, 64 percent were in firms with fewer than 100 employees. About 38 percent of the working uninsured work in businesses with twenty-five or fewer employees.[8] The probability of a firm with fewer than twenty-five workers offering insurance is only .39, compared with .99 for firms with more than 100 employees.[9]

The Growth in Part-Time Employment

Between 1979 and 1988, part-time employment increased 22 percent, and temporary employment increased 164 percent. These employees are less likely to be offered benefits and may be more attractive to employers for this reason. Nationwide, an estimated 38

MANDATED EMPLOYER COVERAGE IN HAWAII

Hawaii has developed three public programs that together provide access to health care to more than 96 percent of the state's citizens. In 1974 Hawaii initiated a policy to ensure health insurance and medical protection insurance for most employees in the state. The nation's only state-mandated employer benefits plan, the Prepaid Health Care Act (PPHCA) requires employers to provide health coverage to their employees. Benefits are basic but substantial, and costs are shared. The employee pays up to 1.5 percent of monthly wages or half of the premium cost, whichever is less. The employer provides the balance, though an employer fund assists employers with fewer than eight employees who need premium supplementation. Small businesses are community rated. Dependent coverage is optional. Two basic plans are available: a fee-for-service plan and a health maintenance plan.

The State Health Insurance Plan (SHIP) was implemented in 1990 to meet the needs of the 5

(continued next page)

percent of the working uninsured work part-time or for only a portion of the year.[10]

The Rising Cost of Insurance

As health care costs have gone up, many employers have responded by reducing benefits, increasing cost sharing, dropping dependent coverage, or dropping benefits altogether. Small employers have been hardest hit by these costs. On average, premiums for small group policies for employers with ten or fewer employees are 20 to 50 percent higher than premiums for policies sold to large employers. Given the marginal nature of many of these enterprises and the low wages of their employees, the cost of insurance may be prohibitive.

The Fracturing of the Population into Smaller Risk Pools

Insurers justify higher premiums in the small group market in order to recoup higher administrative and marketing costs associated with small group business. They also claim that higher premiums are justified because of the greater risk in this line of insurance since there are fewer individuals per employer group over which to spread the cost of a single adverse event (e.g., a premature birth). This concept of greater risk within the smaller group not only increases the cost, but also leads to:

✦ Restrictions on coverage as insurers try to protect themselves against such risk through medical underwriting (i.e., when insurers exclude completely or delay coverage for individuals who are high-risk or have pre-existing conditions);

✦ Redlining (i.e., the exclusion of businesses that are considered to attract high-risk

employees or that, by virtue of the nature of the work itself, such as mining, are considered high-risk); and

✦ Churning (i.e., when insurers opt not to renew policies just at the time when the actuarially calculated risk of increased experience is to occur or the time limit on excluding pre-existing conditions expires).

WHAT ARE SOME APPROACHES TO SOLVING THE PROBLEM?

Within the current system, what options are available to states to help leverage public dollars and to use their regulatory powers more effectively to increase the availability of coverage to the working uninsured? There are four generic approaches states can pursue to assist this population in obtaining health insurance:

✦ Require employers to offer health insurance;

✦ Help reduce the cost of insurance so that it is more affordable;

✦ Directly finance all or part of the costs of care; and

✦ Ensure that the insurance market functions correctly.

These four approaches should not be viewed as mutually exclusive. In fact, if it is assumed that the solution will involve some form of a public-private partnership, then states would have to draw from all four options to craft a workable solution. In addition, these approaches imply a dual role for the state: in some cases the state's involvement would be financial, while in others it would be more regulatory. These new approaches also might require some new roles for the state, including functioning as a reinsurer, marketer, or educator. They also might argue for more innovative uses of existing funds, or the creation of new agencies or the realignment of existing agencies in order for the state to play a more effective role.

A major stumbling block to full implementation of these state options is the Employee Retirement Income Security Act. This federal law preempts a state's power to impose certain changes on self-insured employer health plans. More than 50 percent of U.S. firms are now self-insured. Incentives to self-insure are provided by ERISA, including exemption from state mandates, state-imposed premium taxes, and stringent requirements for financial reserves. These incentives limit the number of employers over which states have authority. Any state solutions to increase access that rely on employer-based insurance cannot depend on the declining number of state-regulated firms.

Require Employers to Offer Health Insurance

The most direct vehicle to ensure that workers have coverage is to require employers to offer health insurance to their employees. This requirement could take two forms. First, employers could be mandated to offer health insurance. Under such a mandate, employers would be required to purchase health insurance for their employees or be subject to a sanction. A mandate approach typically defines the minimum benefits and scope of the health insurance that employers can purchase to avoid the sanction. The sanction could be a civil fine or some other financial penalty sufficient to force employer compliance with the mandate.

Second, employers could be required to either contribute to a public health insurance plan or offer health insurance. This "pay or play" alternative presupposes a state-sponsored public health insurance program. Employer contributions to a public health insurance plan could be based on a fixed dollar amount per employee or based on a percentage of payroll expense. The contribution should be set at a level sufficient to encourage employers to purchase private insurance. Under the pay or play strategy, the amount of this contribution is explicit and, in effect, establishes a ceiling on the employers' costs.[11]

Requiring employers to participate in health coverage makes sense for a number of reasons. Since the focus is on meeting the needs of the working uninsured, it is logical to address this problem at its origin—the workplace. Almost all currently uninsured workers and their dependents could gain coverage if employer requirements were implemented, and if employees were mandated to purchase the insurance provided by their employer.

In addition, this approach could build on the employer-based health care system. No significant changes in the current system would be required. Further, employer requirements create greater equity in the system. Why, for example, should some employers pay for health insurance, while others avoid this responsibility? Employers who offer insurance may be at a competitive disadvantage because of such coverage. Requiring employer coverage thus distributes the responsibility equitably across businesses. It also would help larger employers who currently offer full coverage to improve their competitive position in world markets by reducing much of the cost shifting created by the large number of people without insurance.

(continued from previous page)

percent of Hawaiians falling in the gap between the Prepaid Health Care Act and Medicaid. Under SHIP, the state government subsidizes insurance coverage through a sliding fee schedule for those unable to pay. Insurance companies provide the coverage. Benefits are heavily weighted toward preventive and primary care. However, an individual's hospitalization is limited to five days (two days for maternity). Elective surgery and high-cost tertiary care are excluded. The program assumes that most members of the "gap group" will qualify for Medicaid after reaching the limit for these costly procedures.

SHIP has served more than 12,000 persons in its year of existence, and Medicaid expansions have covered about 5,000 previously uninsured. While these figures demonstrate substantial success, both programs will undoubtedly make additional changes as needed to reach all of Hawaii's uninsured and attain the state goal of universal health coverage. Currently, no change can be made to prepaid health care because of federal restrictions.

Employers who offer good coverage may be increasingly subsidizing the health care costs of other companies through the cost shifting that has taken place in recent years. The growing number of uninsured and underinsured has created a vicious cycle that leaves a smaller number of firms responsible for an ever increasing health care bill. As more people with limited or no coverage enter hospitals or seek physician care, providers are forced to shift their shortfall in revenues from these individuals to patients who have adequate coverage. Physician and hospital charges rise, which in turn pushes up the cost of benefits paid by insurance firms and, thus, the premiums paid by employers. The higher cost of insurance then forces more employers to reduce or drop coverage, further exacerbating the uncompensated care burden on providers and starting the cost shifting cycle all over again.

Employer requirements can help alleviate this problem or even reverse the cycle. By requiring employers to cover their employees, the number of uninsured declines, thus reducing the need to shift those costs. In addition, requirements can establish a minimum level of coverage that can help reduce the number of underinsured. This also will help decrease the need for cost shifting.

Nevertheless, the use of employer requirements also raises a number of concerns. For example:

✦ What size firms will be included? All firms? Only those with twenty-five or more employees? Ten employees?

✦ What exactly will the employer be required to do: Simply offer an insurance product? Pay the full premium? Pay 80 percent of that amount? Pay 50 percent?

✦ What are the benefits that must be included? How much cost sharing? Does there have to be a choice of plans?

✦ To whom must the employer offer insurance? Only full-time workers? If part-time workers are included, how many hours per week should make someone eligible? Thirty hours? Twenty hours?

How these questions are answered may make a significant difference in the feasibility and impact of employer requirements. They help point out some of the difficulties that may be encountered if requirements are enacted. One basic concern—the opposite of the shared responsibility argument—is whether the requirements are too much of a burden on certain businesses. Clearly, to some extent, this is going to be a function of what size firms are included, the portion of premiums paid by the employer, and the treatment of part-time workers.

Since about 50 percent of the working uninsured are in companies with twenty-five or fewer employees, a major concern is that the added financial burden of providing health insurance could be disastrous, particularly for very small or marginally profitable businesses. Any such requirement could lead to higher prices, lay-offs, changes in employee mix (e.g., fewer older employees or females of reproductive age), a shift to part-time employees, and business failures. With regard to part-time workers, it also might lead to a reduction in the number of hours that they can work. For example, if twenty hours weekly were the minimum to be covered under the requirement, then some firms might lower their workers' employment to nineteen hours to avoid the requirement.

A corollary question is whether requirements would be too much of a burden on a state. What impact would they have on tax revenues if businesses are forced to spend pre-tax dollars on exempt benefits? Would firms in a state that requires employer participation move to a state that does not?

The pay or play option affords states an opportunity to address the financial burden of health insurance on employers. The amount of employer contribution to the public health insurance program can be targeted to minimize the impact on all employers or some subset (e.g., by size, profitability, or industry). The state could subsidize the difference between the employer contribution and the cost of the public health insurance program. The issue for a state is the amount of dollars it wants to contribute.

Another potential problem arises from the issue of the employees' share of the premium costs. Many employees would not be able to afford even a small share of those costs. Family income for 35 percent of the working uninsured is below the poverty level, and 85 percent of these working uninsured earn less than $20,000.[12] Even half of a $250-a-month premium may represent too much of a financial hardship to a low-income worker; thus simply mandating coverage may add a burden rather than remove one.

Alternatively, if the employer is required to pay the bulk of the premium, would this not make it more difficult for many small employers to comply? Would it penalize employers currently offering coverage who now pay a smaller percentage of the premiums? Almost two-thirds (64 percent) of employers who offer coverage require an employee contribution for family coverage (43 percent for

employee-only coverage). These employers typically pay only about 60 percent of the premium costs.[13]

Employer requirements may not be sufficient to solve the problems of employees in the so-called redlined industries or those considered high risk. Even if insurance is made available to these groups, its cost may be prohibitive. Or coverage may be excluded or delayed for the very problems for which an individual needs coverage. Requiring open enrollment and community rating may address some of these issues of access and cost.

A final issue regarding employer requirements already has been raised in the context of an argument in their favor: their consistency with the employer-based notion of health insurance that currently forms the basis of the nation's health care system. Employer requirements may be viewed as a logical next step in improving that system. However, some contend that the employer-based system is inherently wrong, and that employer requirements serve only to perpetuate and exacerbate the problems of the existing health care system.

Employer requirements remain an attractive approach to addressing the problem of the working uninsured. On one hand, they have the potential to greatly increase the number of covered workers, create greater equity across employers, and reduce some of the current cost shifting. On the other hand, they also can be inflationary and lead to layoffs. Further, depending on how the requirements are structured, they may not address the needs of the uninsurables and workers in certain industries. If it is assumed that the current employer-based health insurance system is unworkable, employer requirements

WASHINGTON
AFFORDS COVERAGE
TO LOW INCOME

Begun in January 1989, Washington's Basic Health Plan subsidizes premiums for individuals to purchase care from contracting HMOs and PPOs in six cities. The state pays the full premium for those below 75 percent of the federal poverty level. Other enrollees pay on a sliding scale, up to 75 percent of the premium, up to 175 percent of the federal poverty level. The state pays an average of 82 percent of the premium and during the last two years has appropriated about $30 million for insurance subsidies.

Any resident with an income below 200 percent of poverty is eligible for the plan. As of March 1991 the state had enrolled 20,000 individuals. Enrollees receive comprehensive HMO benefits with a $5 copayment for physician visits and no copayment for preventive services. Drug and mental health benefits are not provided. In addition, the plan prohibits medical underwriting, but pre-existing conditions are excluded from coverage for one year.

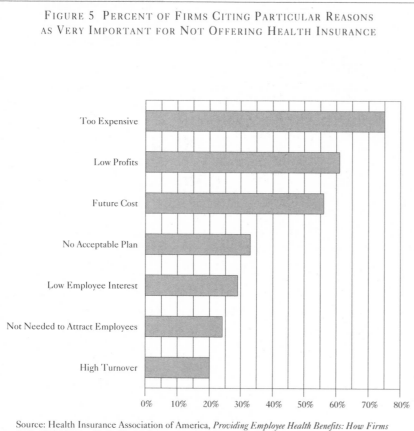

FIGURE 5 PERCENT OF FIRMS CITING PARTICULAR REASONS AS VERY IMPORTANT FOR NOT OFFERING HEALTH INSURANCE

Source: Health Insurance Association of America, *Providing Employee Health Benefits: How Firms Differ* (Washington, D.C.: Health Insurance Association of America, January 1990), p. 32.

◆ Reducing or targeting benefits;

◆ Reducing the cost of health insurance premiums;

◆ Directly subsidizing premium costs; and

◆ Indirectly subsidizing the cost of insurance.

These are not mutually exclusive options. They can be combined in a variety of ways, and together can have a significant impact on making insurance more affordable and available.

Reducing or Targeting Benefits. A controversial issue in most states is whether all insurers should be required to cover certain benefits. These mandated benefit requirements ostensibly stem from a desire to ensure that adequate and comprehensive benefits are available to those who purchase insurance. However, they often also reflect the ability of special interest groups to ensure that their particular specialty or service is paid for.

Proponents of mandated benefits contend that without such mandates, individuals would not be covered for the full range of services they might need. They argue that coverage of benefits such as mental health and substance abuse is as important as coverage for basic medical care, since so many people are in need of those services. Opponents counter that mandating an extensive list of benefits unnecessarily raises the cost of insurance so that it becomes unaffordable to a larger segment of the population. They argue that if low-cost insurance products are to be possible, mandated benefit requirements must be lifted.

Often, these arguments are carried out with more emotion and rhetoric than fact. Available data can be interpreted to support either argument. Studies have indicated that

may exacerbate rather than solve that problem. While requirements ultimately may be necessary, they must be a part of a larger set of reforms that will help correct some of the adverse effects they may create.

Reduce the Cost of Insurance

Even if states require employer coverage, the high cost of purchasing health insurance will continue to make it difficult for many employers and their employees to afford coverage. According to a 1989 survey by the Health Insurance Association of America, the average monthly premium for family coverage was about $250, or more than $3,000 per year.[14] With or without employer requirements, health insurance must be made more affordable (see Figure 5). There are four generic mechanisms to achieve this:

depending on the number of services mandated and the depth of coverage, such mandates will add 3 to 11 percent to the costs of insurance.[15]

Resolving this debate will not be simple. Most would agree that there is a need to cover basic hospital and physician care. However, even this issue is not straightforward. What about high technology and tertiary care? What about preventive and well-person services? Should these types of care be covered? In addition to the issue of which services should be mandated, there is the issue of how much of a service should be covered. For example, should mental health and substance abuse be open-ended benefits, or should there be limits in terms of a dollar amount, number of episodes of illness, or number of units of service?

As states consider these issues, there are a number of basic questions that are important to answer in order to cut through the self-interest and rhetoric that often surrounds the debate:

✦ Is the benefit to be mandated medically necessary and effective?

✦ How much are premiums actually increased by mandating a given benefit? Will this significantly affect the affordability of an insurance product?

✦ Could the benefits required vary for different populations (e.g., younger families may have a greater need for maternity and pediatric coverage, while older families may prefer richer coverage for adult primary care with no maternity or pediatric benefits)?

✦ Is the benefit being offered in its most efficient and effective form (e.g., are inpatient stays better for the treatment of substance abuse than less expensive outpatient modalities)? How much of the benefit is enough?

✦ Is the benefit being managed in terms of medical necessity and appropriateness of service location (i.e., inpatient or outpatient) and frequency of use?

✦ What are the political implications of dropping or adding a benefit?

A number of states already are experimenting with waiving mandated benefit requirements, particularly in the small business and individual markets. These include products now available in Virginia and Washington. These experiments are testing whether more "stripped down" products are of lower cost and are still attractive to the consumer. Unfortunately, it is too early to determine how much of an impact the removal of mandates has had on the small business or individual insurance markets in terms of cost, marketability, or adequacy of coverage.

Reducing the Cost of Health Insurance Premiums. Whatever level of benefits is offered, the high cost of health care is the major reason that health insurance is so costly. Thus, without gaining control over health care costs, it will remain difficult to bring premiums down to affordable levels for many employers and employees.

For more than a decade this nation has tried a variety of incremental approaches to contain the seemingly inexorable rise in health care costs, often with limited success. Costs continue to rise at or above historic rates, and annual increases in health insurance premiums have reached new highs. Clearly, restraining overall health care costs should have a concomitant effect on premium costs and thus the availability of health insurance coverage. There are two major components of health care costs: those associated with the delivery of services and those associated with administration.

Strategies aimed at controlling service delivery costs use managed care as the centerpiece of the effort. While not a new concept, because health maintenance organizations have been part of the landscape since the 1970s, managed care today has taken on new dimensions and meanings. It now is a rubric to describe a variety of activities that emphasize incentives for both providers and consumers to adopt more cost-conscious behavior through the use of negotiated discounts and aggressive utilization review.

Reducing administrative costs is another way to reduce premium costs and thus potentially increase coverage. It is estimated that the administrative costs of the U.S. health care system are almost 25 percent of total expenditures. Comparing this with Canada, where administration accounts for only about 14 percent, suggests that significant cost savings are possible simply by reducing the administrative complexities and duplication inherent in this nation's system.[16]

Directly Subsidizing Premium Costs. The most direct role a state can play in making health insurance more widely affordable is through directly subsidizing the cost of premiums. This can be achieved in a variety of ways, including using employer tax credits, buying down the employees' premium costs, and paying for dependent coverage.

Employer Tax Credits. Employer tax credits are being tried or seriously considered in a number of states, including Kentucky, Massachusetts, Oklahoma, and Oregon. They can

be used in different ways. For example, a tax credit can be made available only to businesses with twenty-five or fewer employees as a means of keeping their insurance costs more in line with larger businesses, which have lower insurance costs. Or a tax credit can be linked to companies that can document that the added cost of insurance would represent too great a financial burden on them. Whatever approach is used, if insurance remains optional to employers, it is important that the tax credit be targeted to those least able to afford insurance for their employees, and not serve as a windfall to employers who have adequate resources to pay for coverage.

Two issues emerge in the implementation of a tax credit, though they apply equally to employee subsidies. First is the question of how much subsidy is enough. On one hand, the credit must be sufficient to make the purchase of insurance attractive to employers. This may vary across employers depending on their size, the nature of their business (i.e., how labor-intensive it is), and the cost of insurance to them. On the other hand, the credit cannot be in excess of what is needed to meet the policy objective. Some market research may be required to determine efficient levels for all of these subsidies.

A second question involves the issue of equity. For example, it is tempting to focus any subsidy only on those who currently do not have insurance. Yet, would that not penalize those employers and employees who currently pay for insurance? Why shouldn't they get the same advantage as employers who have not offered insurance for at least a year? Also, should employers who can afford the cost of insurance but who have simply chosen not to offer it now be entitled to the same tax credit?

Employee Subsidies. Many of the same issues surrounding employer tax credits apply to direct subsidies to the employee. Such subsidies are being tested in a number of states, including Florida, Maine, Michigan, and New York. Employee subsidies can take many different forms. They can involve a flat payment to individuals below some specified income level or they can be based on a sliding scale that is tied to income. Alternatively, they might not involve a specific dollar amount, but could pay for dependent coverage when only the primary wage earner can afford individual coverage. Again, the subsidy might be applied on an income-related basis.

Direct employer subsidies also might be available only to those working in small businesses or to individuals who currently are without coverage. Again, the questions are how much subsidy is sufficient and whether both currently uninsured and insured should benefit equally.

Premium Taxes. Another form of direct state subsidy that can help reduce the cost of insurance is a waiver of the premium tax (i.e., the tax assessed on insured plans). Again, this might be targeted only to small businesses or hard-to-insure industries. This subsidy is not significant enough to solve the problem entirely, since it represents a savings of only about 5 percent, but this form of subsidy can be a part of a larger state strategy. Waiving the premium tax also raises the targeting and equity issues inherent in all direct subsidies.

Employer tax credits, employee subsidies, and premium taxes are not mutually exclusive options, and using them in combination could increase their impact. For example, tax credits to employers can be combined with subsidies for dependent coverage to ensure that employers participate and that an affordable product is available to the entire family. Whatever form of direct subsidy or subsidies is used, it is important to evaluate which has the greatest impact (i.e., makes insurance affordable for the widest segment of the population) for the least state investment.

A number of states are experimenting with a variety of direct subsidy mechanisms. Others are seriously considering moving in this direction. While these demonstrations have proven that subsidies can reduce the cost of insurance and therefore increase its accessibility, they have not yet answered the questions concerning how much is enough and how some equity can be created through the use of the subsidy. What these efforts have demonstrated is the necessity of some form of direct subsidy if the private sector continues to be the principal source of insurance.

Indirectly Subsidizing the Cost of Insurance. In addition to directly subsidizing the cost of insurance for the working uninsured, indirect subsidies might represent effective tools for states. These include reinsurance and subsidization of administrative and marketing costs.

Reinsurance. Reinsurance involves the protection of an insurance company against either a catastrophic event for one of its beneficiaries or expenditures above some agreed-upon aggregate level. Either through the state or a private reinsurance company, the insurer can limit its risk for any claim, or the total costs incurred by a beneficiary under a given contract.

How and why would a state become involved in the provision of reinsurance? Reinsurance can serve a number of purposes. By reducing some of the risk to private insurers, it can decrease their reserve needs and the cost of insurance. It also can serve as a mechanism to help gain access to the market for individuals whom health insurers might consider high-risk or uninsurable. Finally, it can substitute in part for Medicaid by covering some of the costs of care.

A state's involvement in reinsurance can take a number of forms. Most basically, a state can offer some sort of stop-loss coverage above a specified amount (e.g., $25,000). As a means of getting them into the market, this reinsurance could be made available only to small businesses or, initially, to employers who previously have not offered insurance.

One of the arguments that insurers use to explain their lack of interest in insuring small businesses and the high cost of such insurance is their perception of higher risk in small groups. A reinsurance mechanism could, in part, address this concern. By pooling this risk across a large group and reinsuring it, insurers' exposure would be better defined and their costs reduced. In a small group, the potential that currently exists for a catastrophic event makes this market very risky for insurers. A state reinsurance program could make small businesses less precarious and costly, and therefore more attractive to private carriers.

Another form of reinsurance might be directed only at those who are deemed to be high-risk or uninsurable. In this case, individuals would obtain private coverage, but the state's reinsurance program would cover the costs for the conditions that led them to be classified as high-risk. Reinsurance could work in three ways to accomplish this:

✦ As a stop-loss mechanism that would protect the insurer against catastrophic expenses for these groups.

✦ As protection against costs related only to the specific conditions that might make someone a poor risk (e.g., diabetes, heart disease, and high-risk pregnancies).

✦ As part of a contract with designated providers to pay for specific, costly services. Rather than only reimbursing for care, the state could contract with certain designated hospitals that would agree to provide those services either on a discounted or capitated basis. In this way the care might be delivered more inexpensively, the quality could be monitored more effectively, and some form of case management might be made part of the care.

Sources of financing for reinsurance might include existing direct service funding or a new dedicated fund using a hospital or insurance tax, general revenues, or a bond issue. The source of this financing would depend on the level of exposure the state wants to assume, the ability to tap some existing fund, and the population to be covered. For example, if a stop-loss program is initiated for all small businesses, the cost of a reinsurance program would be very high. In that case, it might be financed directly by the health insurance companies, with the state providing seed money to initiate a statewide pool and paying the costs of administering the fund.

What impact would reinsurance have on expanding coverage for the working uninsured? Reinsurance can be an important policy tool for states to use to achieve a number of objectives. First, reinsurance could greatly reduce the cost of an insurance product. It has been estimated that providing stop-loss coverage above $10,000 per year per subscriber might reduce the costs by more than 20 percent. In addition, covering the cost of specified, catastrophic problems will limit the insurers' risk, thereby reducing their reserve needs. The actual savings to the individual will depend on how much of this benefit the carrier passes on in the form of reduced premiums.

A second purpose of reinsurance is to mainstream a larger portion of the population by extending coverage to those who currently may be deemed uninsurable. This would include not only those with serious, pervasive conditions, but also others who are less ill and may not have coverage for some specific condition (e.g., ulcers and heart problems). In this case the reinsurance might help fill the gaps for conditions not covered at all and during waiting periods for pre-existing conditions. It also might make it possible for individuals in the so-called redlined industries to gain access to insurance or lower their cost for insurance. Reinsurance can function as an effective mechanism to help enfranchise segments of the population who otherwise might be excluded. It also may reduce the need to segregate people into high-risk pools that take people out of the mainstream.

In order to mainstream, the linkages between private insurance and the public reinsurance mechanism would have to be more cooperative and specific. Under such an arrangement, the public reinsurance mechanism would reimburse the private carrier once the specified triggers (e.g., stop-loss levels, specific conditions or services, or number of days of institutional care) were met. From the individual's perspective, insurance would thus appear to be a seamless web. All bills would be handled by the private carrier, and individuals would not suddenly be switched from private insurance to public coverage.

Finally, reinsurance provides an opportunity to leverage limited public funds to gain private coverage for a wider segment of the population. In this way it represents a mechanism through which the public and private sectors can establish roles that complement each other, building on their respective strengths.

However, the notion of greater public sector participation in reinsurance is not without risks. The specific role the public sector plays, the potential benefit that can be derived, and the willingness of the private sector to go into partnership with government are outstanding issues. While there are potential long-term benefits to public participation in reinsurance, there is no good track record to draw on. Considerable demonstration of the various approaches is necessary before reinsurance can be viewed as a major part of the solution.

Subsidization of Administrative and Marketing Costs. Another form of indirect subsidy would involve reducing the non-benefit-related premium costs. Small businesses pay higher premiums in part because of the greater costs associated with marketing and servicing their health insurance. On a per member basis, marketing insurance to a large employer is considerably cheaper than trying to sell coverage to a large number of small businesses. These costs include advertising and brokerage fees. In addition, premium collection, which can be done much more efficiently through large employers, also pushes up the costs associated with the small business market. Finally, in large businesses most of the client servicing—including answering questions and helping with claims submission— can be carried out by the employer. This is

FLORIDA SCHOOL DISTRICTS SERVE AS INSURANCE GROUP

A new partnership is being forged between the public and private sectors in Florida. Using demonstration authority granted by the federal Health Care Financing Administration, the state will offer low-cost commercial health insurance through a major Florida school district to families whose children are currently ineligible for Medicaid. The private nonprofit Healthy Kids Corporation, in conjunction with the Florida Medicaid program, will administer the program and subsidize coverage to children in households with incomes below 185 percent of poverty.

Two insurance packages will be offered: a basic plan for preventive and screening services and a comprehensive plan, including inpatient, outpatient, and catastrophic care. Premium payments will be adjusted based on an income-related sliding scale. This demonstration will provide valuable insight into how insurance groups—in this case, children in a specified school district—can be served in creative, alternative ways.

NAIC MODEL
LEGISLATIVE APPROACH

The National Association of Insurance Commissioners (NAIC) has proposed model state statutes to improve the workings of the health insurance market, especially for small businesses. The goals of the NAIC Model Legislative Approach are the following:

Recently Adopted Rating and Renewability Model:

✦ *Address abusive rating practices by limiting the use of claim experience, health status, and duration of coverage as factors in determining ultimate premium rates and annual rate increases for small employers.*

✦ *Restrict cancellation or nonrenewal of coverage provided to small employers.*

✦ *Require disclosure to purchasers of rating strategies and renewal rating factors.*

✦ *Require filing of an actuarial certification and maintenance of*

(continued next page)

much less possible in small businesses, often adding to the costs for the insurer.

The loss ratio is the percentage of each premium dollar that relates to actual benefit payments as opposed to marketing and administrative costs, reserves, and profits. The loss ratio can be more than 90 percent for large groups and can be as low as 60 percent for very small groups. A very good small business product might have a loss ratio of 75 percent. Thus, for the same level of benefits, small businesses might have to pay 20 to 50 percent more.

Some of this difference might be inevitable as long as the insurance system remains employer-based, since it will always be less efficient to reach and serve a smaller group than a larger one. Nevertheless, a state can help reduce these costs by consolidating some of these functions into a single entity that will market and serve insurance products. This can be done directly through a public agency or through support of nonprofit entities in the community that could carry out these functions.

Wherever the organization is located, its functions might include advertising the availability and details of the different products geared to the small business market, initial contacts with and screening of employers, referrals to brokers, and some client services. In this way some of the functions could be made more efficient, brokerage fees could be reduced, and advertising costs could be consolidated.

In states such as California, Colorado, Florida, and Maine, efforts are being made to test this approach. To date these experiments appear to be very promising not only in saving money, but also in helping small employers gain better access to the insurance market.

Given the multiple options and the potential for confusion and even abuse, these entities could be helpful in guiding the small employer through the maze of options. They also could assist brokers in identifying viable leads. Moreover, it might be possible over time to link this support function with some form of pre-certification, which can further assist employers in making the right choices.

Reinsurance and subsidization of administrative and marketing costs are not mutually exclusive options. They can be used jointly or in combination with some form of direct subsidy. In addition to helping reduce insurance costs, they also help the uninsurables gain access to the insurance market, and help make insurance more accessible, understandable, and possibly less perilous to the small employer.

Directly Finance the Cost of Care

Medicaid might be used as a source of direct and indirect subsidies in order to leverage public funds. Alternatively, Medicaid might be extended to cover more directly broader segments of the population. Through a combination of federal mandates and state options, eligibility has been expanded in recent years, and most states are covering an increasingly larger spectrum of the population, particularly pregnant women and children. In some states, including Connecticut, Maine, Minnesota, Rhode Island, Vermont, and Washington, these expansions have gone beyond the federal changes.

Many observers believe these changes in federal law have dramatically altered the traditional, welfare-linked, categorical notion of Medicaid. Federal changes enacted in recent years have greatly expanded eligibility in terms of income levels well above poverty. Moving eligibility up to 185 percent of poverty (about $24,000 in 1990) for some groups has permitted Medicaid to extend coverage to a larger segment of the working population.

Consequently, Medicaid is seen by some as the vehicle through which many of the working uninsured can obtain coverage. However, using Medicaid for this purpose has some limitations. Medicaid is the largest expense in many state budgets. The current pressure on state budgets makes it difficult for states to make even modest expansions in Medicaid. Often, the additional dollars spent on eligibility expansions were balanced by reductions somewhere else, either in Medicaid services or payment, or more likely in other state programs.

If limited public funds are to be used most effectively, one important question is how those funds can better leverage the private system. This can be done through a number of approaches, including subsidies, buying in to private insurance, and reinsurance. While the specific form this participation takes may vary according to a state's needs, the underlying premise is central to any solution: There is a need for the public and private sectors to stop competing with each other, trying to shift the burden and costs. It is imperative for the two sectors to identify how they might best complement each other's role. Short of a completely public solution to the problem of the working uninsured, any viable solution will require such cooperation.

Ensure That the Insurance Market Functions Effectively

Expanding the affordability and availability of private insurance for the working uninsured will place new demands and responsibilities on the private insurance market. New partnerships with the public sector, increased use of community rating, and restrictions on medical underwriting and redlining present new challenges for private insurers and the agencies that regulate them.

Even for insurers who currently are involved in the small business market, there is an understandable degree of caution about expanding that role and entering into new partnerships with the public sector. Many who are experienced in the operation of that market would argue that if reputable private insurers are to expand their role, some basic reform is required to even the playing field and prevent abuses. There is a justified concern that without reform, there is potential for adverse selection and churning. The necessary reforms would have to address the issues of rating, renewals, and underwriting.

Currently, the manipulation of premiums often done to force disenrollment once a subscriber becomes actuarially unprofitable, a lack of guaranteed renewals and other discontinuation practices to achieve the same aim, and abuses associated with medical underwriting and the exclusion of certain industries are detrimental to the success of the small business insurance market. Some companies can cream the market, provide little long-term protection, and reap considerable profit, while leaving more reputable firms with more adverse selection and little motivation to want to stay in the small employer market.

Making this market more equitable and in the best interests of both insurers and consumers would require guaranteed renewals; restrictions on durational rating; and limitations on medical underwriting, pre-existing

(continued from previous page)
certain records to monitor compliance.

✦ *Maintain competition in the marketplace and direct it away from risk selection and toward efficient care management.*

Health Insurance Access Model:
✦ *Ensure access to health insurance coverage, at rates within the limits of the Rating and Renewability Model, for all small businesses, regardless of the health status or claim history of employees and their families.*

✦ *Ensure continuity of coverage for insured small businesses changing carriers and for insured employees (and their dependents) changing jobs.*

conditions, and redlining. Under such reforms, a state could prohibit insurers from arbitrarily dropping coverage for a group. It could require insurers to guarantee the renewal of a policy once it was in effect. In addition, insurers would not be permitted to raise premiums to a point that would effectively force businesses to drop coverage. Finally, businesses would not be arbitrarily redlined as is currently possible, nor would insurers be permitted to exclude so many individuals from coverage because of high health care use or pre-existing conditions. From the insurers' perspective, these reforms might have to be combined with community rating and reinsurance to make them palatable. New York recently has put into place some rules designed to limit abusive discontinuation and renewal practices.

In addition, if subsidies such as reinsurance or the assumption of administrative and marketing costs are provided, there must be some requirement that these savings are directly passed on in terms of reductions in premiums. Finally, community rating or other mechanisms to pool risk across small groups must be encouraged.

ARE THESE EFFORTS ENOUGH?

The working uninsured represent the most significant segment of the population without insurance. While sharing some of the problems generally associated with a lack of insurance coverage, those who work confront additional issues. Solutions to these problems are not simple. Health insurance and the labor market are inextricably intertwined, both in the problems and in the solutions. Consequently, many approaches may have other financial or, in some cases, macroeconomic impacts.

To begin to address these issues will require some new vision, leading to a more multifaceted approach. It also will require discarding some of the traditional roles played by the private and public sectors as well as a redefinition of those roles. Finally, it will require greater regulation of the market, so the market can work freely.

Solutions that require dramatic restructuring should be approached with caution, since each step can have broad, untoward effects. Accomplishing this will require experimentation by states and much greater flexibility on the part of the federal government.

Given the diversity of states, in the end there may not be a single solution. What is important is that the inequities and even the tragedies of the current system can be eliminated and better ways can be found to ensure that those who work and their families have access to comprehensive health insurance.

ENDNOTES

1. Jill D. Foley, *Uninsured in the United States: The Nonelderly Population without Health Insurance* (Washington, D.C.: Employee Benefit Research Institute, 1991), p. 21.

2. Foley, pp. 43, 54-55.

3. Katherine Swartz, "Why Requiring Employers to Provide Health Insurance Is a Bad Idea," *Journal of Health Politics, Policy and Law*, vol. 15, no. 4 (winter 1990), pp. 779-792.

4. U.S. Department of Labor, Bureau of Labor Statistics, *Employer Benefits in Medium and Large Firms* (Washington, D.C.: U.S. Government Printing Office, 1988).

5. William B. Johnston, *Workforce 2000: Work and Workers for the Twenty-first Century* (Indianapolis, Ind.: Hudson Institute, Inc., June 1987), p. xvii.

6. Foley, pp. 46-47.

7. Johnston, p. 59.

8. Foley, p. 49.

9. Health Insurance Association of America, *Providing Employee Health Benefits: How Firms Differ* (Washington, D.C.: Health Insurance Association of America, January 1990), p. 13.

10. U.S. General Accounting Office, *Workers At Risk: Increased Numbers in Contingent Employment Lack Insurance, Other Benefits* (Washington, D.C.: U.S. General Accounting Office, March 1991), p. 4; and Foley, p. 45.

11. The Pepper Commission, U.S. Bipartisan Commission on Comprehensive Health Care, *A Call for Action* (Washington D.C.: U.S. Government Printing Office, September 1990).

12. Foley, p. 35, 54.

13. Health Insurance Association of America, 1990, p. 61.

14. Health Insurance Association of America, 1990, p. 58.

15. Health Insurance Association of America, *Mandated Benefits in Health Insurance Policies* (Washington, D.C.: Health Insurance Association of America, February 15, 1991), p. 9.

16. S. Woolhandler and D. U. Himmelstein, "The Deteriorating Administrative Efficiency of the U.S. Health Care System," *New England Journal of Medicine*, vol. 324, no. 18, pp. 1253-1258.

Building on the Public Commitment

SUMMARY A large number of people are unable to get needed services through employer-based private health insurance. They are vulnerable because of their lack of economic resources, their medical needs, and the barriers imposed by public programs and private insurance.

Medicaid was created to respond to the needs of certain vulnerable populations and is now the most important source of financial access for a wide range of services. In the absence of coherent national health policy, Medicaid has become the vehicle for incremental attempts to expand access, develop new services, and contain costs. States have a huge financial stake in Medicaid, and Governors have used its options to improve coverage and access. States recognize, however, that by itself the program is not the way to ensure access for all those who are vulnerable medically and financially.

States have a number of alternatives, some comprehensive and some targeted to specific populations such as children or the chronically ill. One option is to expand Medicaid to cover more people by increasing the income eligibility levels. Another option is to use Medicaid dollars to purchase insurance or allow people to purchase the services available through Medicaid.

States could establish programs or subsidize the purchase of insurance for certain populations. These options range from establishing a program to cover all children, for example, to providing catastrophic protection for people unable to get private insurance. Another strategy is to expand direct funding of services—not only hospital care, but also clinics and physicians. Finally, states can enhance the voluntary efforts of providers to deliver care to those unable to pay for services. As in other areas of policymaking, there is no unequivocal ideal choice.

WHO IS VULNERABLE?

Of the 34.4 million Americans below age sixty-five who do not have private insurance or publicly financed health coverage, 16.7 percent are nonworking adults and 28.7 percent are children. Of these adults, 58 percent have incomes of less than $8,500 per year. Almost two-thirds are women, and 16 percent are ill or disabled. More than a third of the uninsured children are in families with incomes below the poverty line. Seven of eight children are in families where an adult works full time or part time.[1]

Most children are healthy, though the lack of coverage can mean that they do not get routine care and timely treatment of acute illnesses. For children with chronic conditions, the lack of coverage can impede ongoing management of their condition. Children who have chronic conditions face another problem: While their parents may obtain private health insurance, the child's condition may be exempted from coverage as a pre-existing condition or the child may be medically underwritten and excluded from coverage. For this reason, a large proportion of children with chronic health problems are insured through public programs.

For adults who are not working, coverage may be unavailable. To receive publicly financed health coverage, a person has to meet a strict definition of disability or strict asset and income tests. Like their younger counterparts, adults with chronic conditions frequently lose private insurance coverage because of pre-existing condition clauses and medical underwriting.

THE NONWORKING UNINSURED

+ *66 percent are women.*
+ *30 percent are between age 30 and 44.*
+ *42 percent are at home with family.*
+ *16 percent are ill or disabled.*
+ *15 percent are in school.*
+ *13 percent of uninsured children live in homes where the family head does not work.*

Source: Jill D. Foley, *Uninsured in the United States: The Nonelderly Population without Health Insurance* (Washington, D.C.: Employee Benefit Research Institute, April 1991), pp. 43, 52, 67.

Gaps in coverage for children and nonworking adults ostensibly are filled by public programs. Nowhere is this public commitment more evident than in Medicare and Medicaid. These programs were enacted in 1965 through amendments to the Social Security Act. Medicare provided a new federal program of medical insurance for the elderly and some of the disabled. As a result, coverage for persons above age sixty-five is almost universal.

Medicaid was enacted as a companion to Medicare as the primary source of public health care coverage for low-income individuals and families. And while not all children and nonworking adults without private insurance have access to needed services, Medicaid is an important source of coverage for children and nonworking, nonelderly adults who are poor, disabled, or chronically ill.

HOW DOES MEDICAID HELP?

About 24 million people receive Medicaid—about 10 percent of the total U.S. population.[2] The program serves 10.1 million children below age eighteen and 2.3 million disabled adults between the ages of eighteen and sixty-four.[3]

The program is jointly financed by the states and the federal government. States administer the program under rules and regulations set by the federal government. States are not required to have a Medicaid program, but all states do. Federal rules and regulations establish the basic framework of the program, but states have some discretion in determining eligibility, choosing which services to offer, and deciding how and how much to pay service providers. Because of the variances allowed states, the Medicaid program often is described as fifty different programs.

Medicaid pays providers directly. In almost all cases, those who receive care pay nothing. Eligibility is based on financial and categorical criteria. Medicaid coverage cannot be denied because of medical condition. Finally, Medicaid is the payor of last resort: Public and private insurance must pay for services before Medicaid does.

Medicaid began as a program providing a defined package of services to specified pop-

MEDICAID PROGRAMS IN THE COMMONWEALTHS AND U.S. TERRITORIES

Unlike states participating in the Medicaid program, the federal funding strategy differs significantly for Puerto Rico, the U.S Virgin Islands, Guam, American Samoa, and the Northern Mariana Islands. For these jurisdictions, the Federal Medicaid Assistance Percentage (FMAP)—the rate at which the federal government participates in the funding of the Medicaid program—is fixed at 50 percent. In addition, Congress has established an upper limit on the amount of federal funds that can be used for Medicaid services. In fiscal 1991, the federal limit ranges from $750,000 for the Northern Mariana Islands to $79 million for Puerto Rico.

In light of the fixed FMAP and federal funds cap, Congress gives these jurisdictions more flexibility in administering their programs. Despite the flexibility, they are facing substantial increased costs to administer their programs and must bear the cost solely with their own public funds. For example, in the Commonwealth of Puerto

(continued next page)

(continued from previous page)

Rico, total fiscal 1986 Medicaid expenditures were $143 million. With a federal cap of $63.4 million, federal funds covered only 43.3 percent of program expenditures. It is estimated that total expenditures for fiscal 1990 will be $592 million. Of that amount, federal funds are expected to cover only 13.3 percent of expenditures.

ulations. Today it is the fourth largest source of funding for perhaps the widest array of services available through public programs or private insurance. In 1990 Medicaid funded almost $70 billion in health and medical services[4] (see Table 3).

In the early 1980s Medicaid was the focus of cost containment strategies. From 1982 to 1986, Medicaid expenditures grew at single-digit rates, which was remarkable in the history of the program. However, the success of these cost containment efforts raised concerns that more of the poor were left without access to health care. In response, the program has been expanded in each of the past five years. These expansions now are being reflected in huge expenditure increases. In 1990 Medicaid spending grew by 18.4 percent. Estimated cost increases for 1991 and 1992 are 25 percent and 16 percent, respectively. By 1992 the number of Medicaid recipients is expected to grow by 25 percent. These trends have made policymakers more intent on reforming Medicaid.[5]

Medicaid's growth can be explained in part by changes made to the program since its enactment in 1965. Originally intended to provide access to mainstream medicine for poor women and children and the disabled, today Medicaid provides acute care for women and children; acute care catastrophic coverage; long-term care for the elderly and the physically disabled; and acute and long-term care for the mentally retarded and emotionally disabled. But Medicaid is consistently criticized for not covering all of the poor, forcing people to become impoverished in order to get coverage, not providing all the services needed by each of the eligible groups, and underpaying service providers. Despite these criticisms, Medicaid is the most important source of health care coverage for its intended populations. Moreover, Medicaid's enrollment and costs can be expected to increase due to the growing numbers of uninsured and insurance industry practices, such as medical underwriting and pre-existing condition clauses, that will move more people from private to public coverage. Not all the uninsured would be eligible for Medicaid, and significant gaps in coverage remain.

TABLE 3 MEDICAID EXPENDITURES BY STATE, FISCAL 1990

STATE	EXPENDITURES ($ in millions)	PERCENT OF TOTAL	STATE	EXPENDITURES ($ in millions)	PERCENT OF TOTAL
Alabama	804	1.2	Montana	193	.3
Alaska	153	.2	Nebraska	319	.5
Arizona	553	.8	Nevada	150	.2
Arkansas	618	.9	New Hampshire	226	.3
California	7,047	10.1	New Jersey	2,390	3.4
Colorado	541	.8	New Mexico	294	.4
Connecticut	1,239	1.8	New York	12,187	17.5
Delaware	126	.2	North Carolina	1,499	2.2
District of Columbia	406	.6	North Dakota	199	.3
Florida	2,535	3.6	Ohio	3,262	4.7
Georgia	1,566	2.2	Oklahoma	723	1.0
Hawaii	207	.3	Oregon	537	.8
Idaho	157	.2	Pennsylvania	3,034	4.4
Illinois	2,479	3.6	Rhode Island	446	.6
Indiana	1,487	2.1	South Carolina	857	1.2
Iowa	643	.9	South Dakota	171	.2
Kansas	493	.7	Tennessee	1,439	2.1
Kentucky	1,013	1.5	Texas	3,085	4.4
Louisiana	1,402	2.0	Utah	276	.4
Maine	438	.6	Vermont	154	.2
Maryland	1,182	1.7	Virginia	1,036	1.5
Massachusetts	3,237	4.6	Washington	1,227	1.8
Michigan	2,618	3.8	West Virginia	410	.6
Minnesota	1,472	2.1	Wisconsin	1,482	2.1
Mississippi	624	.9	Wyoming	67	.1
Missouri	948	1.4	**TOTAL**	**69,648**	**100.0**

Source: Health Care Financing Administration, Office of the Actuary, 1991.

Who Is Eligible for Medicaid?

Initially Medicaid was targeted to individuals and families who were eligible for income support programs and, at state option, had high medical bills. Medicaid recipients now can be separated into five distinct populations (see Figure 6):

✦ *Children and Adults Who Receive Medicaid Through Aid to Families with Dependent Children.* This is the largest group of Medicaid beneficiaries, though it represents only 25 percent of total expenditures.[6] Historically, eligibility has been based on meeting the financial eligibility requirements for AFDC, which states determine. Thus, Medicaid eligibility for a family of three ranges from 13 percent of poverty in Alabama to 77 percent of poverty in Alaska.[7] Recent federal legislation expanded coverage by requiring states to cover children up to age six with incomes below 133 percent of poverty and to phase in coverage of older children, up to age nineteen, below 100 percent of poverty.

✦ *People with Physical, Mental, and Developmental Disabilities.* This group comprises about 15 percent of Medicaid recipients, but accounts for the largest share of Medicaid spending—about 38 percent. Twenty-two percent of disabled children and 14 percent of disabled adults are covered by Medicaid.[8] Medicaid coverage is based on income and resources, though income eligibility criteria vary by service and state.

✦ *Poor Elderly Who Need Long-Term Care.* Although only 13 percent of Medicaid recipients are elderly, this population accounts for about 35 percent of total spending.[9] Compared with other Medicaid recipients, the

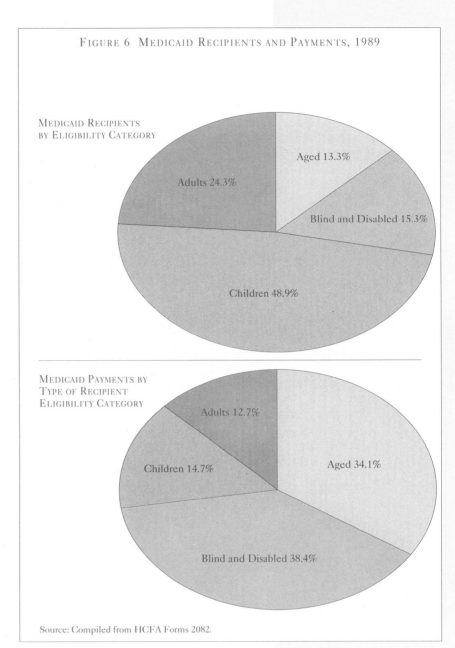

FIGURE 6 MEDICAID RECIPIENTS AND PAYMENTS, 1989

MEDICAID RECIPIENTS BY ELIGIBILITY CATEGORY

Aged 13.3%
Adults 24.3%
Blind and Disabled 15.3%
Children 48.9%

MEDICAID PAYMENTS BY TYPE OF RECIPIENT ELIGIBILITY CATEGORY

Adults 12.7%
Children 14.7%
Aged 34.1%
Blind and Disabled 38.4%

Source: Compiled from HCFA Forms 2082.

elderly disproportionately use nursing home services. The elderly in nursing homes typically are eligible for Medicaid if their incomes are less than 300 percent of Supplemental Security Income (SSI)—about $1,200 per month—or if their medical expenses diminish their income to a specified level, though there are variations among states. Elderly who are not in nursing homes typically become eligible through SSI.

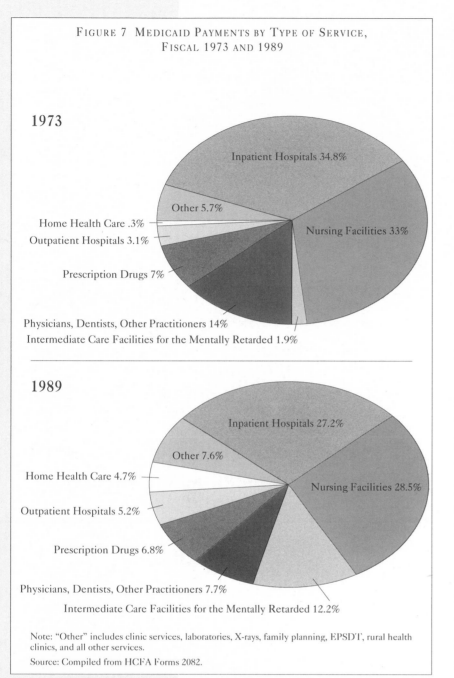

FIGURE 7 MEDICAID PAYMENTS BY TYPE OF SERVICE,
FISCAL 1973 AND 1989

1973

Inpatient Hospitals 34.8%

Other 5.7%

Home Health Care .3%

Outpatient Hospitals 3.1%

Prescription Drugs 7%

Nursing Facilities 33%

Physicians, Dentists, Other Practitioners 14%

Intermediate Care Facilities for the Mentally Retarded 1.9%

1989

Inpatient Hospitals 27.2%

Other 7.6%

Home Health Care 4.7%

Outpatient Hospitals 5.2%

Prescription Drugs 6.8%

Nursing Facilities 28.5%

Physicians, Dentists, Other Practitioners 7.7%

Intermediate Care Facilities for the Mentally Retarded 12.2%

Note: "Other" includes clinic services, laboratories, X-rays, family planning, EPSDT, rural health clinics, and all other services.

Source: Compiled from HCFA Forms 2082.

pregnant women and infants. The historic link between AFDC eligibility criteria and Medicaid was broken. In most states, a pregnant woman only has to show that her income is below poverty and she no longer has to meet the stringent AFDC income and assets tests. Subsequent legislation allowed states to cover pregnant women and infants up to 185 percent of poverty. Twenty-four states now offer Medicaid coverage to these populations between 133 percent and 185 percent of poverty.[10]

✦ *People on Medicare.* Medicaid funds subsidize people on Medicare in two ways. First, some are eligible for Medicaid as well as Medicare because of their income and low resources. Medicaid pays their Medicare cost sharing requirements. Perhaps more important, people eligible for both gain access to Medicaid's comprehensive package of services. Medicare's failure to cover outpatient prescription drugs, a service needed by the elderly and disabled, is the best example of a Medicare gap filled by Medicaid.

Second, Medicaid also pays Medicare cost sharing for people who are not Medicaid recipients. Congress did not want to subsidize the low-income elderly in the face of rapidly increasing Medicare cost sharing, so it mandated that Medicaid provide the financial subsidy. The Medicare Catastrophic Coverage Act of 1988 requires state Medicaid programs to pay Medicare premiums, coinsurance, and deductibles for qualified Medicare beneficiaries (QMBs) with incomes of less than 100 percent of poverty. Subsequent legislation raised the income threshold to 120 percent of poverty beginning in 1995.

✦ *Pregnant Women and Children Who Are Not Eligible for AFDC but Who Have Incomes Below Certain Percentages of the Federal Poverty Level.* This group is the most recent addition to Medicaid. In 1986 Congress responded to the Governors' concern about the high rate of infant mortality by radically changing the eligibility criteria for

Medicaid eligibility is complex. People become eligible for Medicaid in a number of ways depending on their income, assets, age, or condition. Moreover, an individual who is eligible in one state may not be eligible in another. Eligibility also is restrictive. Medicaid eligibility standards disqualify a large proportion of the poverty population. Categorical restrictions make it almost impossible for childless couples or single adults who are not disabled or pregnant to become eligible.

WHAT SERVICES DOES MEDICAID PROVIDE?

The Medicaid program covers a wide range of primary, acute, and long-term care services. Some services are mandatory, including:

+ Inpatient hospital care;

+ Outpatient hospital services;

+ Physician services;

+ Nurse-midwives;

+ Rural health clinics;

+ Early and periodic screening, diagnostic, and treatment (EPSDT) services for children;

+ Family planning;

+ Laboratory and X-ray services;

+ Nursing facility care; and

+ Home health care.

State Medicaid programs also can offer up to thirty-two optional services, such as prescription drugs, respiratory care, and case management. All states offer at least one optional service, and more than half of the states offer more than twenty.[11] The most frequently offered optional services are prescription drugs, services in intermediate care facilities for the mentally retarded (ICF/MR), clinic services, and transportation.

Medicaid offers a comprehensive array of services compared with private health insurance coverage and other public programs. For example, Medicare does not cover outpatient prescription drugs or long-term care. Private insurance policies tend not to cover preventive care, such as well-baby visits and immunizations; long-term care; or specialized services, such as care coordination and residential treatment for the mentally retarded.

The majority of Medicaid dollars go to institutional care, while the majority of recipients use noninstitutional services. In 1990 nursing home care, including ICF/MR, and inpatient hospital care accounted for more than 60 percent of total Medicaid spending. In contrast, the most frequently used services are care delivered by physicians, dentists, and other practitioners; prescription drugs; and outpatient hospital services.[12]

Forty-three percent of Medicaid dollars are used for long-term care (see Figure 7). Medicaid accounts for about half of all nursing home payments, and it is the largest third-party payor for nursing home care.[13] In addition, Medicaid offers personal care, home health care, and an extensive array of medical and social services through special waiver authority. Home health care, waiver services, and ICF/MR were the fastest growing categories of Medicaid spending throughout the last decade. This growth reflects state initiatives to rely less on nursing homes; states are expanding services delivered in the community (including small intermediate care facilities for the mentally retarded) and in beneficiaries' homes. These services include respite care, personal care, home-delivered meals, and case management—all of which can be funded by Medicaid.

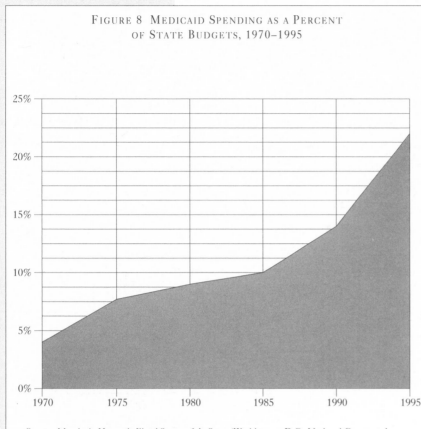

FIGURE 8 MEDICAID SPENDING AS A PERCENT OF STATE BUDGETS, 1970–1995

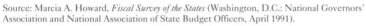

Source: Marcia A. Howard, *Fiscal Survey of the States* (Washington, D.C.: National Governors' Association and National Association of State Budget Officers, April 1991).

States want to increase provider participation, which can improve recipient access to needed services, especially primary care. Efforts aimed at providers have included raising fees, simplifying and streamlining billing procedures, providing additional malpractice protection for obstetrical providers, and establishing provider recruitment programs with state and local physician groups.[14] In addition, states are using new service options for case management and care coordination to oversee service delivery and ensure that Medicaid recipients have access to needed care.

HOW IS MEDICAID FINANCED AND ADMINISTERED?

Financing

Medicaid is financed by the federal government and state governments. Shares are based on a formula that accounts for the per capita income of the state relative to the national average per capita income. States receive federal matching payments ranging from 50 percent to about 80 percent. Nationally, the federal government pays about 55 percent of total Medicaid costs, and states pay the remaining 45 percent.

In 1989 state and local governments spent $27.3 billion on Medicaid—about 14 percent of state expenditures.[15] The National Association of State Budget Officers estimates that by 1995 Medicaid will consume an average of 22 percent of state budgets (see Figure 8). Policy changes at the federal level have great implications for states because Medicaid spending is such a high proportion of state general revenue. Medicaid is the biggest health care program in the states.

The number and types of services covered under Medicaid have expanded since the program's inception. In addition to medical care, Medicaid now offers social and care management services. However, covering a service does not necessarily ensure that it is available. Providers maintain that Medicaid payment rates that are lower than those of Medicare or private insurance hamper access to services. Both payment rates and provider perceptions that non-Medicaid patients do not want to receive care where low-income welfare clients are served contribute to low levels of provider participation in Medicaid. Another concern for Medicaid recipients is the difficulty in getting to physician offices and clinics, which typically are not located near Medicaid recipients' homes.

The financing structure of Medicaid creates strong incentives for expansion. The federal government can expand the program knowing that it has to fund only fifty-five cents for every dollar spent. On the other hand, state governments can expand Medicaid knowing that each dollar of state money can generate one to four dollars of federal money, depending on matching rates. Both levels of government can shift financing for other health programs into Medicaid to control overall budget growth.

Congress' recent spate of mandated Medicaid expansions have severe implications for state budgets. This is especially true during economic downturns, when more persons become eligible for Medicaid just as state revenues are not keeping pace. Thirty-two states expect Medicaid spending to exceed projections in 1991, and twenty-nine states indicate that their revenues will be lower than the estimates used in formulating budgets.[16]

Confronted with mandated expansions and economic crises, states have been forced to reduce spending in the optional components of Medicaid, cut other programs, or find additional revenues. A resolution passed by the Governors in 1990 asked Congress to refrain from enacting additional Medicaid mandates.

Administration

States need flexibility in developing innovative financing and delivery strategies. When given such opportunities, they have moved forward aggressively. Almost all states have taken advantage of federal waiver authority to develop home- and community-based services as an alternative to nursing home care. For example, Oregon has restructured its long-term care service delivery and administration around Medicaid. Most states quickly took advantage of the optional authority to expand eligibility and service options for pregnant women and infants. A number of states have developed sophisticated models for recipient eligibility determination, beneficiary and provider outreach, and service delivery.

At the state level the financing and administration of Medicaid look very different now than in the past. States are coordinating and integrating Medicaid dollars and services with other state programs. Medicaid has become an important contributor to programs in aging, mental health, maternal and child health, education, and public health.

As states address infant mortality, Medicaid services and dollars have been combined with maternal and child health resources to expand services, enroll recipients and providers, and create community support networks in pursuit of a common goal: preventing bad birth outcomes and delivering services to children. Similar strategies are at work in developing alternatives to nursing homes for the elderly and disabled. Medicaid resources have become an important foundation for building state delivery systems.

However, recent federal mandates have limited the opportunities for innovation. These mandates not only take fiscal flexibility away from the states, but also define how states must administer their programs and how states should set priorities for coverage. From the state perspective, more and more of Medicaid dollars and services are becoming uncontrollable and unmanageable.

CONSOLIDATING ADMINISTRATION IN OREGON

Oregon has consolidated all of its long-term care programs into a single administrative structure at the state level and a highly integrated delivery system at the local level. A single state agency, the Senior and Disabled Services Division, manages all of the state's community and institutional long-term care programs. These include Medicaid, home- and community-based services waiver programs, the state-funded Oregon Project Independence, programs under the Older Americans Act, and food stamps and cash assistance for the aged, blind, and disabled. In addition to developing community care systems, the division licenses and certifies nursing homes, reimburses them for the care of Medicaid clients, and develops policies on their participation in Medicaid.

Case management, relocation planning, risk intervention, and pre-admission screening are major components of the service delivery system. These functions are performed by case managers who assess client needs, develop care plans authorizing services, and establish financial eligibility for Medicaid and income maintenance programs.

WHAT OTHER STATE RESOURCES ASSIST THOSE WHO ARE VULNERABLE?

Although Medicaid is the largest and broadest publicly funded program for the low-income uninsured, a wide range of other resources are being used. Together, these programs account for more than 11 percent of total personal health care expenditures.[17]

They include:

✦ *General assistance,* which provides financing for services to the uninsured who are not eligible for any other public or private program.

✦ *Disease-specific programs,* which provide services to persons who have a specific disease or condition, such as AIDS or Alzheimer's disease.

✦ *Subsidies for federal programs,* which supplement federal grant programs beyond state matching requirements (e.g., maternal and child health and social services block grants).

✦ *Medical and social services for the elderly,* which provide home- and community-based services and assisted living arrangements to the elderly who have incomes above Medicaid limits.

✦ *Subsidies to hospitals,* including state appropriations to public hospitals and hospital outpatient clinics, and pool arrangements to subsidize hospitals based on the amount of services delivered to the poor.

✦ *Subsidies to clinics,* including state and local public health department clinics.

✦ *High-risk pools,* which make insurance coverage available to persons who otherwise are uninsurable.

WHAT ARE THE OPTIONS TO IMPROVE ACCESS?

The priority concerns in improving access to health care are the large number of children without health insurance; the problem of access to needed services by the chronically ill, who are small in number but have high medical expenses; and the high dependence of both of these groups on public programs.

Following are six options for improving health coverage for these populations. The options are not mutually exclusive, nor are they exhaustive. All have been tried in some states, and all require that state government take action. The options are:

✦ Build on Medicaid.

✦ Use insurance subsidies to assist selected populations.

✦ Establish state programs for targeted populations.

✦ Provide public catastrophic insurance.

✦ Fund health services directly.

✦ Enhance voluntary efforts.

Build on Medicaid

There are five features of Medicaid that make expansion of coverage through this program an extremely attractive option.

✦ It focuses on the lowest income populations—those assumed to have the least access to insurance and care.

✦ It has a broad benefit package, which provides access to a wide range of services for those with chronic illnesses.

✦ It relies on state administration, which is attractive both because of the low administrative costs and decentralization of program authority.

+ It offers the opportunity to coordinate with other state programs for high-risk populations.

+ It is financed jointly by the federal government and the states.

For all the benefits, there also are significant limitations that make it a less attractive way to expand access. These include the low provider acceptance of Medicaid clients, the "welfare stigma" associated with Medicaid, and the lack of cost sharing, which is appropriate for low-income populations but may lead to unnecessary use of health care services by higher income enrollees.

Proposals to expand Medicaid coverage must consider how to integrate the program with other sources of care. This is important since Medicaid's broad coverage is an incentive for persons to choose Medicaid. Another issue is whether Medicaid could provide transitional coverage for those moving into and out of jobs, or if it could become the primary source of coverage. In addition, the number of providers willing to accept Medicaid beneficiaries must be increased.

A range of expansions could be considered, some extensive, others marginal. Any expansion proposal must address six factors: the people to be covered; income limits; assets and deductions from income; spend-down provisions; benefits; and duration of coverage. Several expansions have been suggested.

Increase Coverage for Low-Income People. Income levels for eligibility have been linked to the AFDC and SSI standards. The new coverage of children, pregnant women, the elderly, and the disabled break these links and establish higher eligibility standards. One option is to take advantage of optional eligibility criteria to apply these higher thresholds to more categories and/or to raise the eligibility standards even further.

Another, more general approach builds on existing categorical definitions of eligibility for Medicaid and the established priority groups. States can ease the eligibility criteria for income maintenance programs, which in turn would make more persons eligible for Medicaid. This would have a large impact on state budgets because more people would receive cash assistance and Medicaid.

Extending Medicaid to higher income individuals will bring in more people who may be able to afford or who have access to private insurance. This is especially true if eligibility is tied to a national standard that does not take into account the differences within and among states. If they remain eligible for Medicaid, recipients have an incentive to keep this coverage rather than taking employer coverage because of Medicaid's comprehensive services and low cost sharing.

Expand Medically Needy Programs. Thirty-seven states and the District of Columbia have a medically needy program that allows those with high medical expenses to become eligible for Medicaid by subtracting their medical expenses from their income.[18] They still have to meet the categorical criteria and the financial resources test. This program has two effects on coverage. First, if the medically needy eligibility level is set above the AFDC level, families with incomes between the AFDC and medically needy standards immediately are eligible for Medicaid. Second, individuals become eligible when high medical expenses reduce their net income and assets below the medically needy level.

Those who are eligible by virtue of high medical expenses have higher per capita costs

NEW YORK'S MEDICAID BUY-OUT

When it has proven cost-effective, New York has opted to pay insurance premiums for Medicaid-eligible individuals with insurance for more than a decade. This means that individuals with $500 net income per month who meet all other Medicaid eligibility requirements can continue to receive coverage through their existing policy and receive Medicaid coverage for services not covered under the policy. Recent data indicate that in 1990 New York paid about $10 million for continued health insurance coverage for 16,596 Medicaid recipients.

In addition to paying the policy premium, the state assumes all responsibilities of that policy, including copayments and deductibles, using Medicaid reimbursements as a guide. To
(continued next page)

than those of the categorically eligible, many of whom are healthy. Medically needy programs reduce the financial burden of costly illnesses.

Use Medicaid Dollars. Some propose that Medicaid funds be pooled for individuals and businesses to buy Medicaid services and to purchase private insurance for Medicaid recipients.

Buy In to Medicaid. This approach would allow individuals, families, and employers to buy Medicaid coverage, much as they would buy private insurance. The premiums for low-income individuals not eligible for Medicaid might be subsidized by the state. A state adopting this strategy would have to obtain approval from the federal government.

States could minimize their subsidy by establishing a premium cost sharing plan to include contributions from the employer and the individual by apportioning either a percentage or a flat amount of the premium. This option might influence employers to encourage their employees to purchase the Medicaid coverage rather than enter the employer's plan. This is especially true if the individual has health problems that will increase the employer's group premium. For example, employers might pay the buy-in premium for their employees. To the extent that an employee's coverage would be provided through Medicaid, rather than the employer's insurance, costs would be shifted from the employer and employee to the state.

Buy Out of Medicaid. States are required to use Medicaid funds to buy private insurance for Medicaid beneficiaries if private insurance is cheaper than Medicaid. This has been done in New York. The state benefits since it pays the average premium for the employer group rather than the full costs of services for the individual. The buy-out option has been advocated to encourage movement from welfare to work, and from Medicaid to employer-based coverage. It also can reduce gaps in coverage when people move in and out of the workforce, increase contracting with managed care plans, and reduce the Medicaid stigma.

From the beneficiary's perspective, the buy-out option has several advantages, particularly reduced welfare stigma and greater continuity of coverage. However, there may be drawbacks, depending on how a plan is structured. Private insurance tends to cover fewer services than Medicaid and it has deductible and coinsurance requirements. For beneficiaries with chronic conditions, pre-existing condition exclusions and other restrictions, such as no prescription drug coverage, also may make the private coverage unattractive.

Buy-out can reduce a state's costs when it shifts a high-risk individual to another group at a premium reflecting average risk. It also can reduce a state's costs if it encourages an individual to take employment and purchase employer-based coverage. On the other hand, it greatly increases the state administrative burden and complexity.

While it may be desirable from the perspective of the beneficiary, buy-out may not offer the state much of a cost advantage and may adversely impact employers. Private insurance premiums are likely to be higher than Medicaid service costs for some Medicaid recipients. It is also likely that private insurance will have higher administrative costs. In these circumstances, private insurance providing the same coverage may be more expensive for a private insurer than under Medicaid. Finally, buying private group insurance through the employer for high-cost cases (e.g., persons with AIDS or disabled children) could greatly increase the premium paid by the employer for the whole group.

In addition to cost issues, most private insurance excludes benefits that support the goals of the Medicaid program. For example, screening children's health is a major goal of Medicaid. Yet such services might not be reimbursed under private insurance. For both cost and benefit reasons, buy-out should be considered as a targeted strategy, where there are particular cost or program goals to be realized, rather than as a general approach to Medicaid reform.

Use Insurance Subsidies to Assist Selected Populations

Another option for states is to establish a subsidized insurance program for selected populations that is separate from Medicaid. These populations could be identified on the basis of income, age, chronic disease status, or other factors. Subsidies could be provided to low-income populations. Such a program can be an alternative to a Medicaid buy-in.

The Washington Basic Health Plan is a model of a state-subsidized program. New York also is conducting several demonstrations of subsidized insurance programs, including separate programs for small employers and individuals. Other states, such as Colorado, Florida, and New Jersey, have similar programs. In addition, Connecticut enacted a separate program in 1990 for pregnant women and children above the Medicaid level and a pilot program for low-income chronically ill adults. However, state financial

constraints will delay implementation of these programs.

One rationale for a program separate from Medicaid is that the needs of the population are different from those of typical recipients, as is this group's ability to pay for care. Thus, a separate program could be constructed with less extensive but more specialized coverage and greater cost sharing than Medicaid.

Separate subsidized insurance programs could be designed to have limited benefits. This limits the cost of the coverage and, in doing so, the extent of the subsidy; and it acknowledges that a substantial amount of care is available from other sources. An incremental program should provide incentives to obtain care that otherwise would be foregone and reduce the financial burden of illness on families.

There are several advantages to a separate subsidized program. However, creating a separate program adds an administrative burden and increases the problems of coordinating eligibility and coverage between this program and Medicaid.

High-Risk Pools. High-risk pools are another form of indirect subsidy in which states might play a role. Twenty-six states have statewide risk pools designed to make private insurance available to persons who otherwise have trouble obtaining coverage because of their health status. The financial risk of covering persons with serious existing conditions or poor health is spread across all insurers in the state (except self-insured employers), who are required to participate in the pool. Persons who have been rejected for coverage by at least one insurance company typically are eligible for the pool. Participants pay a premium

(continued from previous page)

determine whether or not the state will pay the copayment, the physician must first request reimbursement from the insurance company. If the insurance company reimbursement is greater than the Medicaid payment, Medicaid will not make any additional payment. However, if the insurance portion of the bill is less than the Medicaid reimbursement, the state will pay the difference up to the Medicaid level.

Two years ago the state developed a software package to assist in determining the cost-effectiveness of continuing the policy on a case-by-case basis. This new computer system allows the state to collect detailed information on the cost of each case and to determine the cost savings.

that usually is tied to the premium of a small group or nongroup policy. Thus, premiums tend to be high, but not high enough to cover the overall risk of the participant population. Pool deficits generally are subsidized by an assessment on all insurers, though ten states share in this subsidy by granting insurers a dollar-for-dollar tax credit to offset their assessment. Two states, Maine and Wisconsin, subsidize the premium amount for low-income pool enrollees.[19]

High-risk pools can potentially accomplish two important objectives. First, by removing those with high medical expenses from the overall pool, the cost to those who continue to maintain private insurance can be reduced since the remaining risk pool is more homogeneous. However, this will raise the costs for those now in the high-risk pool to prohibitive levels, since their risk is no longer spread across the larger population. Second, for those who are considered uninsurable and thus are excluded from private insurance, the high-risk pool may represent the only source of insurance available to them. During the 1980s, AIDS made the need for high-risk pools particularly evident in some states.

Some argue that high-risk pools defeat the basic purpose of insurance, which is to spread risk over a broad population. Many see a dangerous potential for private insurers to continually narrow the population they cover, shifting more of the burden to the high-risk pool. If the experience some states have had with similar pools for auto insurance is any indication, there is strong evidence to support this reasoning.

Opponents also point to the experience of states where pools currently exist. To date, they have not been entirely effective in protecting large numbers of people, particularly given the high costs associated with them. Less than 3 percent of the uninsured are enrolled in such pools, and it has been estimated that pools typically reach less than 10 percent of those who are uninsurable. Even the most extensive reach only one-quarter to one-third.[20] The low enrollment in these pools suggests that affordability of coverage, not just availability, is a significant issue and that expanding individual coverage to those not in the labor force will require income as well as risk-related subsidies. In many states, making them work would require a state subsidy that might be used more efficiently. However, in the absence of more structural solutions, high-risk pools are considered a necessity in some states as a means of getting some coverage to those most in need of insurance.

Establish State Programs for Targeted Populations

In a large number of states, groups have been actively promoting the creation of universal unitary insurance programs. These would provide coverage for the entire population under a single plan administered by state government.

Several arguments can be advanced for a universal program for children. Children are a priority within society. Most would agree that children's access to health care should not depend on their parents' income. Children are relatively healthy, so such a program would have relatively low cost. A substantial number already are insured through public programs, including many of those who need the most expensive care.

Similarly, several arguments can be made for a universal program for the nonelderly who are severely chronically ill but not totally and permanently disabled. This is a relatively small population, so the aggregate costs of their care would be relatively low. A special insurance program might address their needs, including prescription drugs and effective case management, better than standard insurance. Insurer efforts to avoid insuring this population have contributed to the crisis in the small group and individual insurance markets.

Still another potential population to whom universal coverage could be extended is pregnant women. The country is seeking to reduce infant mortality by expanding prenatal care, and there is a clear consensus on the appropriate standard of care, so benefit requirements are clear.

Provide Public Catastrophic Insurance

An alternative to broad-based public insurance is public catastrophic coverage, which would be available for high-expense illness. There are at least three approaches states can take:

◆ Offer catastrophic insurance policies that could be purchased by individuals or companies.

◆ Create catastrophic expense programs in which the state pays for all or part of the costs of care above a specific amount.

◆ Provide reinsurance or stop-loss protection for insurers.

Each proposal needs to be evaluated in terms of its impact on access to care, family finances, and provider finances; its acceptability to individuals and families; and its costs.

Catastrophic Coverage. One option is for government to provide catastrophic insurance coverage. Such coverage would have high deductibles, and copayments also could be required.

It is likely that catastrophic coverage policies would have little impact on access to care. They would not pay for most routine or ambulatory care and therefore would not encourage people to get care when symptoms first appear. However, once a family met the catastrophic deductible, its access to covered services would be enhanced.

The impact on family finances may be substantial. In particular, catastrophic coverage could preserve the resources of families confronting high-expense illness. Those who would benefit the most would be the middle- and upper-income populations who otherwise cannot obtain insurance.

Public acceptance of catastrophic health insurance policies is not clear. They are not widely available or widely purchased. A hybrid catastrophic/primary care policy developed in Colorado has been found to have market appeal. Called SCOPE, this policy pays for preventive services in full, while physician office visits require a $15 copayment. For hospital inpatient care, enrollees must pay a $250 deductible and half of the first $5,000 in charges. The state's Medical Indigency Fund will help pay costs for low-income enrollees using participating hospitals. Coverage against high total out-of-pocket expenses, together with low deductibles and high copayments, could be more attractive than true catastrophic coverage.

(continued from previous page)
Eligible people are those below the age of sixty-five who, nine months prior to application, have been rejected from private health insurance coverage due to a medical condition; have had their coverage so drastically limited in scope as to be useless; or have had their premiums increased by more than 50 percent. There are no financial qualifications for membership, and about 10,000 people are enrolled. The plan offers a comprehensive benefit package. There is a six-month pre-existing condition clause. The state rate-setting board sets the premium rates, which cannot exceed 150 percent of the standard health insurance rate. Enrollees must meet a $1,000 deductible and a 20 percent copayment on all costs up to $5,000. There is a $500,000 lifetime maximum.

State Catastrophic Expense Programs. During the 1970s, four states—Alaska, Maine, Minnesota, and Rhode Island—created catastrophic expense programs. These programs sought to limit the impact of uninsured and costly illnesses on families. Only Rhode Island's program is still operational. The other programs were discontinued because they served few people at a relatively high cost per person served.

Established in 1975, the Rhode Island program covers catastrophic expenses and provides substantial coverage for mental disorders and heart disease, and prescription drugs for the elderly. The program also addresses uncovered services of insured patients. To encourage insurance coverage, the program has a lower threshold for those who also are insured. In 1988 more than 95 percent of those served by the program were insured, including 70 percent by Medicare.

A few other states are experimenting with programs. New York has a demonstration catastrophic expense program. New Jersey has established a program for catastrophic expenses for children below age eighteen.

Catastrophic expense programs have been seen as a way to protect people from the high costs of care. They have not built effective political constituencies, largely because so few benefit from them.

State Reinsurance/Stop-Loss Protection. A third approach to catastrophic coverage is for the state to serve as a reinsurer of individual insurance policies. Under this approach, the state would reimburse insurers in cases where claims exceeded a set amount. The state would subsidize the costs to the insurer of this reinsurance or stop-loss protection. Sup-

porters believe that the subsidy would encourage insurers to again offer individual insurance policies and to offer lower rates to high-risk individuals. It would reduce the level of medical underwriting.

This proposal can be compared with commercially available reinsurance. While reinsurance is available commercially, premium costs are based on the population covered. If the pool is small and high-risk, as it is likely to be, the reinsurance premiums will be high. Subsidies would reduce premiums.

There are two potential drawbacks to this mechanism. Higher income individuals are most likely to benefit from the subsidies, since they are more likely to purchase individual coverage. Second, by reducing the risk borne by the insurer, the state creates an disincentive for the insurer to monitor or control the costs under these policies. This can be reduced if the insurer retains some risk even for very high-expense cases.

Fund Health Services Directly

Much of the current health care for the uninsured and underinsured is financed by grants and appropriations directly to providers. Direct federal and state funding of services is substantial. In 1987 federal, state, and local programs paid an estimated $45 billion for personal health care services other than Medicaid and Medicare. State and local governments paid $21.5 billion, or nearly 50 percent. In addition, state and local governments spent another $13.1 billion on public health activities, including some personal health services.

The bulk of the state and local funding was to provide care in hospitals ($14.1 billion), while physician services constituted $4.1 billion, nursing home care $600 million, and drugs and sundries $400 million. These funds supported public hospitals; payments to private hospitals for programs such as maternal and child health; public health clinics; community health centers; and programs to address the needs of specific populations, such as the special supplemental food program for women, infants, and children and McKinney Act programs for the homeless.[21]

One option for states is to expand direct funding of services, especially outpatient services. This approach could fund a wider range of services. Another advantage is that funds could be used for outreach to hard-to-serve populations, such as pregnant teenagers or the homeless, who otherwise might not seek care.

There are disadvantages to the service strategy. These programs are more vulnerable to budget cutting than entitlement programs, such as Medicaid. Second, funding specific providers restricts freedom of choice, and in some cases, directs people to "charity" care. Third, some areas, including rural areas, may need substantial investments in physical plant or provider recruitment to put capacity in place.

The traditional models of direct service delivery rely on hospitals or organized clinics. Alternatives have been developed that may be suitable where public health clinics do not exist or where they are unprepared to provide general health services. In Fairfax and Chesapeake, Virginia, for example, the county governments contract with physicians to provide a specific number of visits at a reduced charge or no charge. These visits are coordinated by county staff. Other network models could be developed.

Enhance Voluntary Efforts

Both physicians and hospitals provide care at a reduced charge or no charge to indigents. This care is financed through direct philanthropy and through cost shifting. States can consider actions to reinforce and standardize these voluntary care systems. Efforts could be made to improve coordination of voluntary activities, strengthen providers' commitment to serve the poor, and create programs to share the burden more equitably.

Improve Coordination of Voluntary Activities. The Kentucky Medical Society and Fairfax (Virginia) Medical Society have a program in which physicians provide a certain number of visits per week at no charge. They also have a system for matching acutely ill individuals with physicians. A coordinating physicians group within each society solicits the participation of additional physicians and publicizes the program.

Strengthen Provider Commitment to Serve. This may be done in several ways. Licensing acts may specify that hospitals must provide services without regard to an individual's ability to pay. Some states require hospitals to provide a minimum level of charity care or community service to be eligible for tax-exempt status. Other states require physicians to accept Medicare assignment or be prepared to accept Medicaid patients. Reasonable and relevant standards and effective systems for monitoring compliance are critical to the success of these approaches.

TEXAS COUNTY INDIGENT HEALTH CARE PROGRAM

The Texas County Indigent Health Care Program (CIHCP) was established in spring 1985 under the Indigent Health Care and Treatment Act. CIHCP is a county-administered program designed to provide health care for the poorest Texans, who are inadequately insured or without health insurance. Counties without public hospitals or hospital districts must establish programs and set aside 10 percent of their general revenue tax levy to pay for services. CIHCP counties that expend more than 10 percent receive state matching dollars for the excess expenditures. Inpatient and outpatient hospital care, skilled nursing care, physician services, prescription drugs, and laboratory, X-ray, and family planning services must be provided.

In state fiscal year 1990, 142 Texas counties had active programs. About 11,700 household applications were approved for services, with an average household size of 1.5. CIHCP counties expended $24.8 million for services, and the state government provided another $1.4 million. About 60 percent of the expenditures were for hospital-based care.

The voluntary care system relies on cross-subsidies—cost shifting—to a significant degree. As the market for hospital services becomes more price-sensitive, hospitals that have to substantially mark up their charges to subsidize charity care may be at a disadvantage compared with hospitals having smaller charity loads. To address this issue, some states, including Florida, New Jersey, New York, and South Carolina, have created indigent care pools.

Under these arrangements, all hospitals contribute a percentage of their net revenues to the pool. The funds are distributed back to hospitals in proportion to their efforts to serve the poor. Florida's pool has been used to fund Medicaid expansion, and New Jersey and New York have used their pools to fund a variety of demonstration projects. These pools have been criticized as "sick taxes," but since they pool funds from insured patients, they are as broad-based as the funding streams that pay the insurance premiums.

Are These Strategies Sufficient?

Two conclusions regarding the options are especially noteworthy. First, Medicaid is a major source of coverage for the nonworking population. To a large extent, the options presented here can be characterized as expanding Medicaid, building parallel insurance programs to Medicaid for selected populations, replacing Medicaid (and other insurance programs) with a broader plan, or supplementing Medicaid with direct services. In each of these cases, the strengths and weaknesses of the state's Medicaid program need to be considered, and integration and coordination between Medicaid and the option under consideration is a critical concern.

Second, some of the options are expanded entitlement, some are subsidized insurance products, and some are expanded direct services. Entitlement offers the least control over spending and the least targeting, but greater assurances of access. Direct services offer the greatest control over costs and greatest targeting to those most in need, but the highest risk that access will be cut through budget reductions or failure of growth to match inflation. As in other areas of policy-making, there is no unequivocal ideal choice.

Endnotes

1. Jill D. Foley, *Uninsured in the United States: The Nonelderly Population without Health Insurance* (Washington, D.C.: Employee Benefit Research Institute, 1991), p. 68.

2. U.S. Department of Commerce, Bureau of the Census, *Statistical Abstract of the United States: 1990* (Washington, D.C.: U.S. Department of Commerce, 1991), Table 2.

3. Foley, pp. 21, 52.

4. Health Care Financing Administration, Bureau of Data Management and Strategy, HCFA Forms 2082, 1989.

5. Health Care Financing Administration, 1989.

6. Health Care Financing Administration, 1989.

7. National Governors' Association, "State Coverage of Pregnant Women and Children," *MCH Update* (Washington, D.C.: National Governors' Association, January 1991), p. 12.

8. B. Griss, *Access to Health Care*, vol. 1, no. 4 (Washington, D.C.: World Institute on Disability, March 1989).

9. Health Care Financing Administration, 1989.

10. National Governors' Association, *MCH Update*, p. 11.

11. Health Care Financing Administration, Office of Intergovernmental Affairs, *Medicaid Services by State* (Washington, D.C.: Health Care Financing Administration, 1990).

12. Health Care Financing Administration, 1989.

13. Health Care Financing Administration, 1989.

14. Deborah Lewis-Idema, *Increasing Provider Participation: Strategies for Improving State Perinatal Programs* (Washington, D.C.: National Governors' Association, July 1988).

15. Marcia A. Howard, *Fiscal Survey of the States* (Washington, D.C.: National Governors' Association and National Association of State Budget Officers, April 1991).

16. Howard, 1991.

17. Helen C. Lazenby and Suzanne W. Letsch, "National Health Expenditures, 1989," *Health Care Financing Review*, vol. 12, no. 2 (winter 1990), p. 11.

18. National Governors' Association, *Catalogue of State Medicaid Program Changes* (Washington, D.C.: National Governors' Association, 1990).

19. R.R. Bovbjerg and C. Koller, "State Health Insurance Pools: Current Performance, Future Prospects," *Inquiry*, vol. 23 (summer 1986), pp. 111-121; B. Griss, *Access to Health Care*, vol. 1, no. 3 (Washington, D.C.: World Institute on Disability, December 1988); B. Griss, 1989; and Jeffrey C. Merrill, *State Initiatives for the Medically Uninsured*, Annual Supplement, HCFA Publication No. 03311 (Washington, D.C.: U.S. Government Printing Office, December 1990).

20. Griss, 1988, 1989.

21. Jack Needleman, Judith Arnold, John Sheils, and Lawrence S. Lewin, *The Health Care Financing System and the Uninsured* (Washington, D.C.: Lewin/ICF, 1990), pp. 75-77.

Managing Costs Incrementally

SUMMARY   As the second largest purchaser of health insurance in the nation, states are affected by the dramatic growth in health care costs in two ways. First, they purchase health care through Medicaid and other state-funded public health programs. Second, they purchase health benefits for their employees. Because of their purchasing power, states command considerable leverage in the health care market. Within the current system, opportunities exist for states to use their position and influence to control rising health care costs.

Specifically, states can:

✦ Use managed care to promote cost-effective provider and patient behavior;

✦ Use their buying power to secure discounts in the purchase of employee health care;

✦ Reduce the impact of cost shifting by making coverage available to more people; and

✦ Make better use of existing regulatory cost containment tools.

While these incremental cost containment strategies are useful, their long-term impact in controlling costs is limited. Thus, these strategies cannot be considered a substitute for structural reform of the health care system.

WHAT IS THE STATE ROLE IN FINANCING HEALTH CARE?

States are the nation's second largest purchaser of health services, after the federal government. They purchase about 7 percent of all health care provided in the United States. In 1991 states will spend about $8 billion for state employee health benefits and almost $40 billion for persons covered under Medicaid.[1] Many states also have general assistance programs covering low-income persons ineligible for Medicaid and sponsor a number of indigent care and targeted health programs (e.g., maternal and child health programs).

For these reasons, states are well positioned to negotiate favorable discounts for health services with organized systems of care. By becoming prudent purchasers of care, states can demand greater value for their health spending in the form of utilization management, volume discounts, and efficient delivery of health services. In fact, many of the lessons learned by private industry in containing health costs can be applied successfully by states.

HOW CAN STATES REDUCE HEALTH CARE SPENDING?

States can employ four strategies to control health care expenditures incrementally. First, states can use a range of managed care interventions. These efforts are focused on the populations and providers covered under state health programs, particularly employee benefit plans. Second, states can use the buying power derived from their large employee base to effect substantial discounts. Third, states can reduce the impact of cost shifting on the cost of care. Finally, states can make better use of existing regulatory cost containment tools.

Each of these approaches holds considerable promise for incremental cost reductions in state health care expenditures, either by reducing health care costs or by protecting the state from inequitable cost shifting by other payors. However, the approaches are less promising for sustained control of the long-run rate of increase in health care costs. Thus, while states can make considerable gains in reducing their expenditures in any given year—an important and worthwhile goal—technology advances and rising labor costs are likely to continue their upward pressure on the rate of health care cost increases. This will continue to affect the full range of payors.

Use Managed Care

"Managed care" is a term covering a wide range of utilization and reimbursement control strategies designed to limit costs and improve the quality of care. Managed care attempts to contain costs through a combination of aggressive negotiation, review of utilization for appropriateness and effectiveness, and incentives for providers and patients to limit costs. Although managed care typically is known as a means of promoting cost-effective utilization of health services, negotiated provider discounts represent a large share of the potential savings under these programs.

Managed care strategies are implemented through organized systems of care designed to promote the cost-effective use of health services by modifying the behavior of both providers and patients. Provider behavior is modified through the creation of networks of providers who agree to practice according to some notion of "medical appropriateness"

under predetermined reimbursement arrangements. Patient behavior is modified through benefits program designs that encourage patients to obtain care through the provider network where utilization can be reviewed and controlled.

Provider Network Options. Central to most managed care strategies is the creation of organized provider networks with systems of utilization review and/or financial incentives that promote the cost-effective use of health services. The provider exchanges a discount in charges and some autonomy in the practice of medicine for increased patient volume. The states' ability to deliver a large volume of health purchasers to individual providers greatly strengthens their ability to establish such networks.

Influence over costs and practice patterns can be maximized in exclusive contracting arrangements such as health maintenance organizations (HMOs). Employers pay a fixed premium directly to the HMO, which is then responsible for meeting the health needs of covered beneficiaries. Although HMOs differ, HMO physicians are either employees of the plan (staff model) or a partnership of physicians (group model) who typically serve only HMO beneficiaries. The capitated nature of HMO premiums creates an incentive to minimize costs by emphasizing cost-effective medical practice. Also, a physician's income in HMOs typically is linked to a profit-sharing plan, which provides additional incentives to limit costs.

An HMO also can deliver care through networks of providers known as an independent practice association (IPA). An IPA is an association of physicians who agree to provide services at negotiated rates in exchange for increased patient volume. Several reimbursement mechanisms are used with IPA physicians, including fees for service, capitated amounts per patient, and risk-sharing arrangements. IPAs typically are used with benefit plans that provide financial incentives for individuals to access the provider network. IPA physicians also have an incentive to avoid unnecessary utilization because carriers often monitor utilization to favor networks that minimize costs.

The IPA model may be less effective in influencing physician practice patterns than the staff and group model HMOs because health plans generally do not have an exclusive arrangement with IPA physicians. IPA physicians often belong to several IPA networks and usually treat non-network patients, and the diverse clientele of IPA physicians limits the ability of any one plan to influence provider behavior. It is generally believed that the more exclusive a plan's contracting arrangement with providers, the more effective the plan will be in promoting cost-effective medical practice.

Utilization Controls. Most managed care systems include varying degrees of utilization control designed to discourage unnecessary or ineffective treatment. Utilization controls include a range of procedures that permit the health plan to review the choice of treatment, either prospectively or retrospectively, to encourage cost-effective medical practice. There are several types of utilization controls that can be applied before, during, or after care is provided (see *Utilization Management Strategies*). Although utilization controls generally are applied to both network and non-

network providers, they typically are most effective in networks where incentives for physicians to comply with cost controls are greatest.

Many conventional health plans require that the patient or physician's office consult with medical personnel employed by the carrier before certain classes of nonemergency procedures are performed. Known as precertification, this approach permits the purchaser to consult with the physician to ensure that the procedure is medically necessary. Although these utilization controls typically apply to hospitalizations, increasingly they are being applied to certain outpatient surgical procedures and high-cost diagnostic tests. Many insurers also require second opinions to avoid unnecessary health expenditures in cases where alternative treatments are available. Nearly 75 percent of all workers are in plans with some type of precertification requirement, and 66 percent are in plans requiring second surgical opinions for a select list of nonemergency procedures.[2]

Utilization controls also can be applied both during and after the point of service. Many plans monitor hospital stays with discharge planning, case management (typically for high-cost cases), and concurrent length-of-stay review. Many plans retrospectively review individual claims to determine the appropriateness of utilization, identify inconsistencies between medical records and hospital bills, detect errors and fraud, and identify candidates for case management. In some networks, reimbursement is denied for tests and procedures deemed medically unnecessary.

Utilization controls are predicated on notions of appropriate medical practice. Stan-

Pre-Service Strategies

Precertification Program requiring prior determination by a payor's agent that proposed medical services are appropriate for a particular patient.

Second Surgical Opinion Program requiring a patient to obtain an opinion about the appropriateness of a proposed treatment from a practitioner other than the one making the original recommendation.

Referral Controls Program in which a primary care physician or gatekeeper coordinates, manages, and authorizes all health care services provided to a covered beneficiary.

During-Service Strategies

Case Management A process for identifying potentially high-cost patients and facilitating the development and implementation of less costly and more appropriate courses of care.

Concurrent Length-of-Stay Review An evaluation initiated during a patient's hospitalization of both the appropriateness of admission, for emergency admissions that could not be reviewed through prior authorization, and the need for continued hospital stay.

Discharge Planning Identification of a patient's health care requirements and arrangement for the provision of services after discharge from the hospital.

Post-Service, Pre-Payment Strategies

Medical Policy Edits Based on standards of proper medical care, information presented on a hospital or physician claim is reviewed, and a determination is made about whether the claim should be paid as presented.

Central Medical Review Assessment by medical staff employed by the insurer of claims that were suspended by the claims processing system or resubmitted by beneficiaries or physicians for additional review.

Procedure Code Review A process by which claims are reviewed for correct coding by physicians. Code review software identifies and either recodes or suspends the claims for which the codes have been incorrectly used.

Post-Payment Strategies

Hospital Bill Audit Hospital bills are checked for billing and payment errors, as well as for appropriateness of itemized services. The focus usually is on large-dollar inpatient or outpatient hospital bills.

Medical Record Review Review of medical record data to determine the appropriateness of a particular course of treatment.

Retrospective Claims Review Statistical review of paid claims data to identify providers and beneficiaries with notably different patterns of health care utilization.

Fraud Detection Identification of fraudulent billing as submitted by hospitals, professionals, other providers, and insurance claims personnel.

dards of medical appropriateness typically are based on statistical averages of regional medical practice adjusted for individual circumstances. Over time, these standards are likely to be modified to reflect recent efforts to develop practice guidelines. These guidelines are based on ongoing research on the appropriateness of alternative procedures under various conditions.

These practice guidelines have been used in some managed care systems to help physicians avoid unnecessary procedures and improve medical outcomes. Some of these guidelines have been incorporated into managed care systems with automated procedures used to assist in the precertification process. It is estimated that costs have been reduced by roughly 3 percent in places where practice guidelines have been incorporated into the precertification process.[3]

Benefits Design Models. Managed care plans usually are coupled with a benefits design that encourages enrollees to obtain care through the desired provider network where utilization and cost controls can be applied. For example, plans typically offer favorable cost sharing (i.e., lower copayments) as an inducement to obtain care through network physicians. The stronger the incentive for individuals to access the network, the more effective the managed care plan will be in containing costs. In fact, the effectiveness of a managed care plan can depend on the extent to which the benefits design encourages patients to use network providers.

Health benefits design has emerged as one of the most controversial issues in employee compensation. Strong financial incentives to access network providers often are viewed by workers as restrictions on their freedom of choice in selecting providers. The issue is so inflammatory that many employers have weakened incentives for workers to confine their care to network physicians. This may be a particular concern in states where state employees are represented by well-organized unions or associations that are capable of exerting influence on the legislative process.

Largely due to the controversy over restrictions in freedom of choice, benefits designs vary substantially across plans. Benefits designs range from lock-in arrangements, under which individuals are covered only for care provided by a network physician, to complete freedom of choice. Lock-in arrangements are most prevalent in HMOs where care is provided only by HMO physicians (unless a patient is referred to a non-HMO specialist), and inpatient care is provided only in hospitals designated by the HMO. As an inducement to enroll in a lock-in plan, enrollees may enjoy lower cost sharing than is typically found in conventional health plans. The lock-in model provides maximum control over utilization for covered individuals.

Most managed care plans have adopted benefits structures that fall somewhere between the lock-in and complete freedom-of-choice models. Enrollees in these plans typically choose their provider but are rewarded with favorable point-of-service cost sharing if they use network providers. For example, many plans have established preferred provider organizations (PPOs) where cost sharing and balance billing are eliminated for patients who use network physicians. Others offer reduced cost sharing for persons accessing the network (e.g., cost sharing of 10 percent for network providers and 20 percent for other providers).

Benefits packages also can be structured to provide incentives for individuals to comply with various utilization controls. For example, patients may face a penalty for failing to comply with precertification requirements. Plans also may deny coverage for specialty care unless a patient first obtains a referral from a network provider. These referral controls, which are designed to eliminate unnecessary specialty care, are most effective in capitated plans such as HMOs.

Managed Care in State Employee Health Plans. Most states have incorporated some managed care strategies into their employee benefits plans. About forty-two states offer an HMO; in eight of these states more than half of the state workers are enrolled in an HMO.[4] Nationally, about 29 percent of state workers were enrolled in an HMO in 1990, down from 32 percent in 1988. Half the states have preferred provider organizations in place where state employees are encouraged to use a PPO network through reductions in cost sharing.

Most state plans also include some form of utilization control. More than 80 percent of state plans require some form of precertification, and second opinions are required in thirty-eight states.

The Role of Managed Care in Containing Costs. Managed care plans are capable of producing cost savings. Many in the insurance industry believe that HMOs can reduce costs by 10 percent or more, and many large corporations and state governments can point to decreased dollars spent on health care with the advent of managed care plans. There is some expectation that the potential for cost savings under managed care will grow as medical effectiveness and outcomes research

are developed. Despite its promise, the cost-effectiveness of managed care systems is not indisputable.

Much of the current savings is considered marginal or occurs one time only. Managed care plans are unable to limit underlying health care costs related to technology development and dissemination. Plans will be forced to spend money as these costs rise. Moreover, managed care programs often are burdened by high administrative costs for both the plan and providers, which offset any potential savings. Finally, HMO premiums tend to shadow those of indemnity plans, and there is little evidence to suggest that HMO fees fairly reflect the cost of providing care.

Not all managed care plans are equally effective. Due to their organizational structure, the more loosely arranged plans such as PPOs show little if any overall savings. It appears that managed care is most effective in modifying medical practice when network providers serve exclusively those covered under the plan (i.e., the HMO model), and when patients obtain their care exclusively through the network. Unfortunately, these optimal conditions are not always achievable given the multitude of practice options available to physicians and the public demand for freedom of choice in providers.

Use the State's Buying Power

As large as state employee plans are, their bargaining power could be enhanced by consolidating state, local, and city employees into one purchasing entity. By expanding the plan to include municipal employees, including school system employees and public utility authority workers, a state could as much as triple the number of persons represented in the consoli-

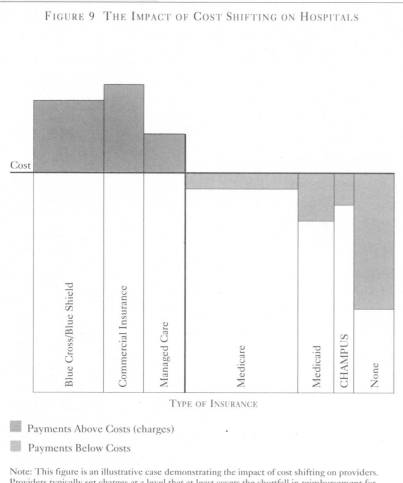

FIGURE 9 THE IMPACT OF COST SHIFTING ON HOSPITALS

Cost

Blue Cross/Blue Shield

Commercial Insurance

Managed Care

Medicare

Medicaid

CHAMPUS

None

TYPE OF INSURANCE

■ Payments Above Costs (charges)

■ Payments Below Costs

Note: This figure is an illustrative case demonstrating the impact of cost shifting on providers. Providers typically set charges at a level that at least covers the shortfall in reimbursement for persons who are uninsured, underinsured, or covered by public programs. An increase in uncompensated or undercompensated care costs must be accompanied by an increase in charges above costs to meet provider operating costs.

Source: Lewin/ICF, 1991.

the open market, thereby increasing the per capita cost in the plan. This would increase state health benefits costs if the state's premium is keyed to per capita costs. States could protect themselves from these cost increases by basing state costs on the actual experience for state employees.

Including Medicaid enrollees would greatly increase the volume of services in the plan. However, state employee unions may resist this approach. Moreover, some states might need to increase reimbursement for Medicaid enrollees to attract providers. Because the geographic location of Medicaid recipients differs from that of state workers, this may limit the impact on the state's bargaining leverage. However, this approach could be used to broaden access for Medicaid enrollees by requiring physicians to treat Medicaid patients as a condition of network participation.

Reduce the Impact of Cost Shifting

Providers attempt to recoup uncompensated or undercompensated care costs by increasing overall charges for services (see Figure 9). Such cost shifting has increased in recent years due to increases in the uninsured population, reductions in covered benefits, and efforts by payors to negotiate discounts.

Like other purchasers of health care, states pay for health care to the uninsured and underinsured by shifting costs. Moreover, some states pay directly for the uninsured population through state appropriations to public hospitals and other health care facilities and programs. Thus, states stand to share in the potential cost savings of incremental strategies for reducing the impact of cost shifting through alternative financing of health care for the uninsured.

dated bargaining unit. This would greatly enhance the state's bargaining leverage to effect substantial volume discounts. The effectiveness of this strategy depends on the number of participants in the plan and the concentrations of state and local employees in particular geographic areas. In many areas of a state, the number of state and local workers may be too small to effect substantial discounts.

Permitting small employers to become part of the plan also could help broaden a state's purchasing power. However, broadening representation also may attract higher risk groups who have difficulty obtaining insurance on

Several factors need to be considered in determining whether incremental efforts to reduce cost shifting will result in net savings to the state. First, many of the existing approaches for reducing uncompensated care rely to some degree on state appropriations, raising the possibility that contributions from the state treasury will outweigh potential savings in state employee premiums. Of course, where the state has decided to participate financially in the solution to the problem, this may be an acceptable trade-off.

Second, some incremental strategies are designed more to redistribute the cost shift than to actually reduce the cost shift amount. This distinction is an important one. For example, some provider tax and pooling arrangements may do little to reduce the statewide cost shift amount because hospitals as a group must still cover the cost of the provider tax in their prices. Thus, the pooling ameliorates the uneven distribution of uncompensated care among providers—an important goal—but continues to generate an overhead charge for insurers and employers.

Third, because people lack health insurance for a variety of reasons, any one approach to expanding insurance coverage is likely to affect only a portion of cost shifting. For example, high-risk pools address only the small proportion of the uninsured who have been denied coverage because of an existing health condition. Moreover, an estimated 30 percent of uncompensated hospital care nationally will be unaffected by any strategy to expand coverage because it is generated by insured patients who fail to pay for uncovered services or copayments.[5] Also important is the extent to which reductions in cost shifting will actually be converted into premium savings for the state. Some observers have argued that hospitals are unlikely to pass along savings from reduced cost shifting and that insurers are unlikely to convert the savings into reduced premiums absent other cost control interventions.

Finally, there is the issue of one-time savings versus durable cost control. Like the other incremental strategies, efforts to reduce uncompensated care may result in one-time savings to the state, but leave unabated the underlying rate of increase in health care costs.

Provider Taxes and Revenue Pooling Arrangements. Several states rely on a hospital tax to raise revenues for indigent health care initiatives, often pooling the money with other revenue sources to redistribute and reduce the uncompensated care burden among hospitals. Hospitals typically are assessed a specified percentage of net patient revenues. The funds often are then combined with other revenue sources and used to finance indigent care programs or provide direct support to hospitals with high indigent care burdens. Some states have considered extending this so-called provider tax to physicians and other ambulatory care providers.

States have turned to provider taxes as a financing mechanism because of their inability to apply taxes or surcharges across all insurers. Under the Employee Retirement Income Security Act, states are prohibited from regulating a range of employee benefits, including employer-sponsored health insurance. States can impose a tax on commercial insurers as a way of raising revenues for care of the uninsured, though all employers who self-insure or provide employee coverage without using a commercial insurance company to pool the risk are exempt from the tax. Many large employers are self-insured, reducing substantially the amount of insurance that can be taxed. To circumvent ERISA, many states have established provider taxes with the goal of spreading the financial burden across all insurers (including the self-insured) through higher provider prices.

The purposes of state pooling arrangements vary. Some are designed primarily to raise revenues. For example, Maine taxes hospitals in order to subsidize its insurance risk pool for uninsurables and to pay the administrative costs of the state Health Care Financing Administration. Other pooling arrangements are more explicitly aimed at redistributing uncompensated care burdens. In New York the rate-setting system includes regional charity care pools designed to distribute the burden of unpaid care among hospitals. In Ohio, South Carolina, Virginia, and Wisconsin, where hospitals would otherwise face a competitive disadvantage if they served an inordinate number of indigent patients, the tax is designed to equalize the financial burden. Several of the provider tax and pool arrangements also are used to finance other health care initiatives such as local primary care programs.

Whether provider tax and pooling arrangements result in savings to the state depends on the structure of the arrangements. When a federal Medicaid match is involved, significant new dollars are brought into the system and employers, including states, can potentially reduce cost shifting. However, new state expenditures also are involved in Medicaid spending. In addition, there is some risk in using the Medicaid matching strategy because the federal Health Care Financing Administration is expected to issue regula-

tions that may limit the use of provider taxes for Medicaid.

Without federal Medicaid dollars or some other nonstate contribution to the pool, direct savings to the state are less likely. This is because the tax and pooling arrangement alone may redistribute uncompensated care but do little to actually reduce it. Redistribution can be very important in a broader effort to contain costs through competition, but direct savings to the state are likely only if the state is subsidizing indigent care in particular hospitals that stand to gain more from the pool than they contribute (e.g., state public hospitals).

Expanded Employer-Based Insurance. A number of states have considered requiring all employers to participate in providing insurance, either through a mandate or through pay or play arrangements. Another approach is to make insurance more affordable for employers who currently are not purchasing insurance. California, Massachusetts, and Oregon are testing the use of tax credits. Moreover, the Robert Wood Johnson Foundation currently is sponsoring a series of demonstration projects that are designed to make insurance more affordable by pooling or subsidizing administrative costs, tailoring benefits, and obtaining substantial discounts from providers. Many states are involved in these demonstrations, often contributing subsidies from general revenues.

Employer-based approaches to insurance expansion can have some impact on cost shifting, though there are important limitations. First, nationally less than 30 percent of hospital uncompensated care results from uninsured workers and their dependents. The remainder stems from insured persons, for noncovered benefits and unpaid copayments, and nonworkers. Although these proportions vary among states, they demonstrate the importance of coverage for nonworkers as well as for the employed population. While it is true that many of the adult uninsured are working, roughly 25 percent are unattached to the labor force, and another 22 percent are part-time or seasonal workers who are unlikely to receive insurance benefits regardless of employer benefit policies.[6]

Employer-based strategies tend to reach only a small proportion of uninsured employees. For example, several of the Robert Wood Johnson demonstrations have seen substantial enrollments in recent months, but the numbers are small compared with the number of uninsured. Even with subsidies and lower premium costs, many employers continue to be unable or are unwilling to purchase insurance. Enrollments through the tax subsidy programs also have been relatively small to date, though experience with these programs is still relatively new.[7]

Expanded Insurance Coverage for Individuals. States also can consider incremental methods for expanding insurance coverage more directly to individuals—for example, through high-risk pools. These approaches can be aimed at both the employed population without insurance and those who are unattached to the labor force.

State Requirements for Blue Cross/Blue Shield Plans. Four states require Blue Cross/Blue Shield plans to offer nongroup coverage with open enrollment and no age adjustment of premiums. In eight other states, the plans traditionally have offered open enrollment as a general practice. Open enrollment provides an opportunity for persons who otherwise would be regarded as uninsurable to obtain

coverage regardless of pre-existing conditions, and serves as an alternative to a state high-risk pool. Blue Cross/Blue Shield open enrollment policies provide coverage to a broad mix of high-risk populations and tend to make nongroup premiums more affordable.

State-Subsidized Nongroup Insurance. Hawaii, New York, and Washington have implemented state-financed insurance plans aimed at both working and nonworking populations ineligible for Medicaid. The plans generally are available on a sliding scale basis to persons below 200 percent of the federal poverty level. The New York plan, which is part of the state's broader Regional Pilot Program for the Uninsured, subsidizes existing plans purchased through private carriers. The other plans are offered directly by the states. All of the plans require substantial state financing, but they also rely on premium payments by beneficiaries, thereby bringing some private dollars into the system to help offset uncompensated care.

The potential for these individual insurance approaches to reduce uncompensated care varies. Risk pools focus on the small proportion of the uninsured with existing medical conditions. However, because individuals in this subpopulation are more likely to be hospitalized, they could represent a relatively high share of uncompensated care attributable to the uninsured. Yet very low enrollment rates in most of the states with high-risk pools have limited their potential impact on uncompensated care costs. These low enrollment rates have been attributed to the high price of premiums despite subsidization, as well as a lack of outreach and advertising in most of the states.[8]

THE NEW JERSEY HEALTH CARE TRUST FUND

Comprehensive reform legislation recently enacted in New Jersey will make health care more affordable for state residents. A major component of the Health Care Cost Reductions Act is the Health Care Trust Fund that replaces the Uncompensated Care Trust Fund. The new fund, which will be used to pay for uncompensated care, is financed through a tax on all the bills of paying patients. The revenues collected through this tax are paid to the state monthly and appropriated to Medicaid, allowing New Jersey to receive federal matching funds. This program is expected to generate anywhere from $250 million to $300 million per fiscal year.

(continued next page)

Other approaches either lack evidence or enough experience to demonstrate a measurable impact on uncompensated care. However, as with the other incremental approaches, they focus only on the segment of the population that is generating uncompensated care.

Medicaid Eligibility Expansion. Probably the most expedient method available to many states for reducing uncompensated care is Medicaid expansion. Available federal matching funds vary between 50 percent and 80 percent of total program costs. States also can offer direct coverage for the uninsured through general assistance or general relief welfare programs, but these are fully financed with state dollars.

Some states already have maximized Medicaid eligibility by covering all populations allowed by the federal government on an optional basis. Others can still add populations without increasing costs in the associated cash welfare programs, Aid to Families with Dependent Children and Supplemental Security Income. It is likely that the "medically needy" option will have the greatest impact on uncompensated care. This is because it allows certain persons to obtain Medicaid coverage if they incur large enough medical bills to "spend down." These persons have too much income to qualify for cash assistance but become eligible for Medicaid if their income drops below income eligibility thresholds once medical bills have been subtracted. Thus, many large hospital bills that otherwise are generating uncompensated care can be covered by Medicaid and its attendant federal match.

Make Better Use of Existing Regulatory Cost Containment Tools

The 1980s were a paradox of dramatic increases in health spending and diminished access to care. The number of persons without health insurance increased substantially, while national spending for health services grew at more than twice the rate of inflation. Rising costs have made health insurance less affordable, which has contributed to reductions in insurance coverage, increased uncompensated care costs, and a growing reliance on state and local indigent care programs. Cost containment must be an essential element of any program to expand insurance coverage and could prove vital to maintaining even the existing level of access.

Most states have adopted some form of regulation to limit the growth in health spending, though cost containment typically is only one objective of these approaches. Regulators are charged with balancing the often contradictory objectives of discouraging expansion of high-cost, inefficient facilities and promoting access in underserved areas. Regulators also must attempt to limit health spending while promoting high-quality health care. The tension created by these competing objectives often is at the heart of controversies over the effectiveness of these regulatory approaches.

Control of Capital and Technology. About forty states have a program called certificate of need (CON) to limit the expansion of hospital and nursing home facilities and control the diffusion of new technologies. CON is a regulatory review process that requires certain health care organizations to obtain prior authorization from the state before making major capital expenditures, purchasing some high technology equipment, or offering new or expanded services. Although CON provides a forum for controlling costs through resource planning, it has been criticized as excessively litigious and ineffective.

The Purpose of Certificate of Need. The primary purpose of CON has been to reduce systemwide health care costs by preventing duplication of facilities, delaying the diffusion of new technologies, and encouraging cost-conscious renovations of facilities. CON also is used to promote other health policy objectives such as expanding access to care by promoting and protecting institutions that care for underserved populations; fostering community involvement in the development of health services; and encouraging service and facility development that conforms to state and regional plans. Moreover, by incorporating quality indicators into the approval process, CON can be used to promote high-quality health care (see *Certificate of Need Objectives* on p. 83).

Although CON programs vary by state, they generally require that project developers demonstrate a need for proposed projects as a precondition for CON approval. "Need" is defined by specific criteria established by law and regulation. Quantitative measures often are used to demonstrate conformance to CON criteria, including projected utilization rates, bed need formulas, and the extent of services provided in a given geographic area. Many states also include in their CON programs licensing requirements that limit the provision of certain high-cost services to facilities meeting minimum standards of patient volume, state training, and quality of care. States also may require facilities to provide a minimum level of charity care to be licensed to perform certain procedures.

The Controversy Over CON. Critics of CON argue that it has failed to contain the growth in hospital spending and actually may have increased costs by protecting inefficient providers. They argue that competitive markets can determine the appropriate levels of capital investment better than regulatory agencies. The CON process also has become very litigious, which has substantially increased the cost of regulation to all parties.

Another criticism of CON is that the process often is very politicized and vulnerable to special interests. In some cases, highly publicized debate over CON applications actually has accelerated the diffusion of technology by elevating public perception of the minimum levels of services that should be available through local providers. This can result in inefficient resource allocation, increased costs, and diminished quality of care. In recent years concern over the effectiveness of CON has led several states to discontinue their programs.

The Impact of CON. The rates at which CON applications are approved or denied generally are considered poor measures of program effectiveness. While high approval rates may suggest a lenient process, they also may reflect a tightly controlled program with well-articulated goals and criteria that deter applications. The best way to evaluate CON is to analyze the experience of states with and without CON programs in slowing the rate of growth in health spending. There are several studies on the impact of CON on hospital facilities, technology and services, and nursing homes.

✦ *Hospital Facilities.* As a cost containment measure, CON is premised on the theory that excess capacity invites increased hospital uti-

(continued from previous page)
Another important cost containment measure is the development of a state health plan that determines approval of certificate of need applications. In addition, the minimum filing fee for certificate of need was increased from $1,000 to $5,000 and the limit on nonprofit hospital liability was raised from $10,000 to $250,000. The bill also prohibits health care practitioners from referring patients to services in which they or their family members have a financial interest.

The new legislation also enacts initiatives to improve access. A Health Start Plus program provides prenatal, obstetrical, and social services to pregnant uninsured women and infants with incomes between 185 percent and 300 percent of poverty. The act also makes available $6 million for insurance pilot programs for small employers.

lization, particularly in a third-party payor system that renders consumers insensitive to cost. Seeking to maximize occupancy and lacking incentives to reduce admissions, providers will attempt to increase utilization of facilities. Thus, eliminating excess capacity is seen as a means of slowing the rate of admissions and limiting the growth in health spending.[9] Although the literature indicates a correlation between capacity and rates of admission, no causal relationship between the two has been demonstrated.[10]

Critics of this theory point out that capital expenditures are a relatively small component of hospital costs and that restrictions on capital are unlikely to reduce costs unless coupled with utilization controls. The majority of studies conclude that CON does not slow the increase in costs,[11] and studies that do show savings report them to be small.[12] Some studies suggest that costs may have increased under CON due to anticipatory or anticompetitive effects. For example, some researchers have shown that eliminating small low-cost hospitals, such as those found in rural areas, can increase costs by shifting patients formerly treated in these facilities to higher cost hospitals.

✦ *Technology and Services.* Growth in technology is widely believed to be one of the primary reasons for rising health care costs, and restricting the availability of technology could theoretically be expected to slow the increase in health spending. However, studies of the effect of CON on the diffusion of technology are divided on the program's impact. While some studies show that CON can control the expansion of certain technologies, such as CAT scanners,[13] others have shown that it has failed to limit the availability of several surgical procedures.

Limiting the diffusion of technology through CON has proven difficult. Due to the strong public demand for the latest in life-saving technologies, the CON approval process often becomes so politicized and emotionally charged that it is difficult for regulators to impose limits.[14] Also, there are several administrative difficulties in controlling new technologies, particularly in cases where these services are provided through independent vendors who are not under the jurisdiction of the CON regulatory process.

✦ *Nursing Homes.* Evidence indicates that CON does constrain both total nursing home costs and the supply of nursing home beds. Occupancy rates in nursing homes average about 92 percent nationwide, suggesting that further restrictions on nursing home construction can be expected to reduce overall costs. However, studies reveal that the demand for nursing home beds exceeds the number available, suggesting that CON has limited access to nursing home care.

CON controls on the number of nursing home beds directly affect state spending for institutional care under the Medicaid program. For example, because few persons have long-term care insurance, an expansion in the number of nursing home beds ultimately would increase the number of people eligible for Medicaid. Restricting the supply of nursing home facilities is thus a means of controlling expenditures under the state's Medicaid program. A number of states, including Oregon and Wisconsin, have established a moratorium on nursing home bed expansion to redirect these resources to home- and community-based services.

Regulation of Provider Reimbursement. Several states and the federal government have attempted to contain the growth in health care costs by regulating the amount charged by providers. The federal government has limited the increase in hospital reimbursement for Medicare patients through its prospective payment system (PPS). In addition, several states have established mandatory hospital rate-setting commissions.

CERTIFICATE OF NEED OBJECTIVES

Moderating Cost

CON was intended to limit capital investment by preventing the addition of unneeded services and facilities; reviewing major renovations or buildings to encourage providers to be more cost-conscious and limit expenditures not related to need; restricting overspending on needed projects as well as preventing unnecessary projects entirely; and limiting the proliferation of expensive new medical technologies, restricting them to settings and amounts deemed to be efficient.

Promoting Access

CON has been used to protect providers of care to underserved groups, particularly providers serving indigent and geographically isolated populations. Methods used include disallowing the addition of new facilities that attract private-paying patients away from providers in underserved areas; favoring provider applicants with a proven commitment to the care of indigent patients; limiting service closure in geographically isolated areas and restraining expansion in more populated areas; and predicating CON approval on the condition that specified levels of service are provided to the underserved.

Fostering Community Involvement in Capacity Development

CON has been used to promote the involvement of communities in the development of health care services. Community involvement permits the development of health programs tailored to the particular requirements of a given population. Community support gives political clout to decisionmakers who find it difficult to determine which services should be made available.

Encouraging Development That Conforms to State Health Plan Goals

Because states determine the criteria by which CON applications are judged, they can formulate criteria to encourage the advancement of state health plans. States can use CON to promote the availability of increasingly intensive health care services through a hierarchy of facilities distributed across an area (the regionalization of health care). States also can use CON to influence the location and character of new facilities or predicate the availability of a new service on appropriate use of that service and its relationship to disease prevention.

Promoting Quality

Although CON was never intended to monitor the quality of care provided, quality indicators can be incorporated into the approval process. Also, CON can positively influence quality by requiring that certain high-risk procedures be both subject to oversight by an inhouse standing review committee and conducted under the supervision of staff possessing specified educational and professional credentials.

As an alternative to rate regulation, many states have emphasized expanding competition among providers as a means of containing the growth in health costs. For example, many states have encouraged exclusive contracting and regulated discounts, or have required public disclosure of hospital rates to inform consumers and encourage price competition among providers. Recent studies indicate that states emphasizing competition have been about as successful as regulated states in slowing the growth in health spending. The debate over competitive versus regulatory approaches has intensified as the rate review process has become increasingly litigious and politicized.

Hospital Rate Setting. While several states have some form of hospital rate regulation, only four states are considered to have comprehensive rate-setting systems. Maryland, Massachusetts, New Jersey, and New York regulate rates for all non-Medicare payors. Until recently, all four had Medicare PPS waivers that permitted them to regulate hospital rates for Medicare patients. Maryland currently is the only state that still has a Medicare waiver, making it the only true "all-payor" system in the nation. However, the other three states are still considered to have all-payor systems because they regulate rates for all non-Medicare payors.

The primary objective of rate setting is to restrain the growth in hospital costs. By limiting the growth in reimbursement levels, hospitals are given an incentive to become more efficient, resulting in fewer admissions and shorter lengths of stay. The all-payor system also facilitates programs for pooling uncompensated care costs across all hospitals so that no single provider is unfairly disadvantaged in providing a disproportionate share of charity care. As with CON, however, rate regulators face multiple and potentially conflicting responsibilities such as containing costs while preserving quality, and maintaining the financial stability of hospitals while ensuring access in underserved areas.

The methods used in setting rates vary by state. In some states rates are set on either a per diem or a per case basis, such as in the diagnostic related group (DRG) system used in New Jersey. In other states only aggregate hospital revenues are regulated, giving the hospital the freedom to vary rates across payors. Rate-setting states use adjustments for case mix, but beyond that there is no adjustment for the intensity of care required for individual patients. This is a particular concern for smaller rural hospitals, where the care of one or two very expensive patients per year could result in costs substantially greater than the revenues allowed under the rate-setting system.

Rate setting can be used to reduce cost shifting among payors. For example, all payors in Maryland, including Medicare and Medicaid, pay the same rate, thus eliminating the cost shift arising from undercompensated care and negotiated provider discounts. However, not all states set uniform payment rates for all payors. In fact, there is some concern that states can use rate setting to promote cost shifting for Medicaid patients.

Impact of Rate Regulation on Costs. Most studies of rate regulation indicate that it has been successful in slowing the rate of increase in hospital spending. The evidence generally shows that in rate-setting states the rate of growth in hospital expenses per admission is lower than the rate observed in unregulated states.[15] However, the experiences of individual states differ. Some regulated states have experienced above-average increases in hospital spending, while hospital spending in many nonregulated states has been increasing at rates well below the national average.[16]

Studies also show that rate setting has been more successful than CON in controlling the rate of increase in hospital spending.[17] One reason is that rate-setting decisions directly affect revenues, whereas the relationship between CON approval and cost is much less clear to both regulators and the public. Rate setting deals directly with current payment amounts, while CON has only indirect effects on hospital rates, most of which will not be apparent for several years. Also, rate regulation has been implemented in states with high hospital costs and where the motivation to contain costs has been strong.

Criticisms of Rate Regulation. Critics argue that rate setting eliminates incentives for providers to innovate and can result in a general misallocation of resources. According to this argument, when states adopt rate setting, hospitals are transformed from private institutions competing on the basis of price and quality into regulated utilities maintained for the public good. Due to the politicized nature of the process, regulators will have incentives to sustain inefficient hospitals that otherwise would have closed. Moreover, critics argue that the loss of competition reduces incentives for efficiency and can slow innovation in the delivery of health services. The process also has become increasingly litigious, which can raise the cost of regulation to all parties.

As an alternative to rate regulation, several states have attempted to contain costs by promoting price competition among providers. For example, in 1982 California enacted legis-

lation permitting plans to negotiate contractual arrangements that would channel beneficiaries to selected providers, usually in exchange for a discount in price. Several states also have promoted managed care and provider networks in order to contain costs by promoting competition among providers on the basis of price and quality. The effectiveness of this approach in containing costs compared with regulation remains unclear.

Reimbursement Controls for Nonhospital Services. Until recently, rate regulation has focused primarily on inpatient hospital care. Hospitals were the logical place to initiate rate regulation because they account for more than 44 percent of all health spending and are less difficult to regulate than the thousands of physicians practicing in each state. While rate regulation has slowed the growth in hospital spending, it has accelerated the growth in ambulatory care costs, as services formerly provided on an inpatient basis have been shifted to outpatient settings. In response to these rapid increases in ambulatory care costs, beginning in 1992 Medicare will regulate physician charges with fee schedules based on the Resource Based Relative Value Scale.

Proposals now are emerging at the state and federal levels that would establish all-payor fee schedules and expenditure targets for all physician services in an effort to contain the growth in ambulatory care costs. The major problem with physician fee schedule models is that while they limit the fee per unit of service, they do nothing to control the volume of services provided. In the face of declining reimbursement, some physicians may attempt to compensate for the loss of income by increasing the volume of services prescribed for patients. Studies show that in

SELECTIVE PROVIDER CONTRACTING IN CALIFORNIA

In 1982 California established a program to purchase hospital care services provided to Medi-Cal beneficiaries. Under the Selective Provider Contracting Program (SPCP), the state contracts with hospitals that want to discount the cost of their services for the care of Medi-Cal beneficiaries. In return, when a sufficient number of hospitals in a geographic area agree to participate in the program, the remaining nonparticipating hospitals are no longer eligible for reimbursement for services to Medi-Cal beneficiaries, except for emergency care. The state was granted a freedom-of-choice waiver from the federal Health Care Financing Administration so Medicaid beneficiaries also could be served under the program.

As of January 1991, 237 hospitals participated in SPCP—a sufficient number to provide all inpatient care under Medi-Cal. The state estimates that it has saved about $400 million for fiscal 1990.

Canada, which has physician rate controls, physicians perform more procedures per patient than in the United States.

Perhaps the greatest concern with physician rate setting is its impact on innovation and the quality of care. Critics argue that under rate-setting systems, physician income is decoupled from the quality of care provided. Because fee schedules do not vary with physician performance, innovative physicians will earn as much as those who are less entrepreneurial. It is argued that reductions in the financial incentives to excel in the delivery of health care could have significant implications for the quality of care provided and the quality of individuals entering the profession.

Tort and Medical Liability Reform. The rapid rise in health spending has been fueled in part by an increase in the size and frequency of medical malpractice lawsuits. The rise in medical liability claims has increased medical malpractice insurance costs and increased the practice of defensive medicine. In some cases medical liability costs are so great that many providers have reportedly changed specialties, contributing to a shortage of physicians in obstetrics and certain surgical specialties.

Like other forms of tort liability, medical malpractice is governed by state law. Many states have enacted reforms designed to reduce costs and counter the adverse effects medical liability has had on access and provider practice patterns.

Medical Malpractice Costs. The rapid rise in medical liability costs is largely attributed to growing public expectations of the health care system. Widely publicized advances in technology and the potential size of malpractice awards have elevated public expectations. Critics of the current legal environment also point out that the potential size of malpractice awards has encouraged both plaintiffs and attorneys to pursue frivolous claims. Moreover, patients increasingly attempt to hold providers responsible for poor health outcomes even in cases where there is little evidence of negligence by the physician.

The process of determining negligence often is subjective. Providers generally are considered negligent if they deviate from standards of accepted medical practice. However, standards of accepted medical practice often are unclear and inconsistently applied. Moreover, the demise of locality rule (i.e., the use of local practice standards in determining negligence) has brought national medical standards into local communities.[18] This has made it easier for medical experts from outside the community, potentially those with questionable expertise, to influence malpractice proceedings with their own individual interpretations of accepted practice.

Medical malpractice costs also can be affected by the subjective nature of awards. In a successful malpractice claim, the plaintiff may receive an award covering real damages such as loss of income and continuing care costs; compensation for pain and suffering; and punitive damages often intended as retribution or a deterrent to further malpractice. Real damages can be determined on the basis of measurable economic losses. However, pain and suffering and punitive awards are subjectively determined, which often results in inconsistencies.

Perhaps the most costly consequence of the growth in malpractice claims has been the practice of defensive medicine. Fear of malpractice litigation reportedly has caused providers to overprescribe certain tests and procedures to protect themselves in the event of a lawsuit. The problem is said to be particularly acute in obstetrics, where there has been a sharp increase in the number of cesarian births and increased reliance on fetal heart monitoring.[19] Critics argue that these practices have added to health care costs with only marginal improvements in health outcomes.

Containment of Malpractice Costs. States' efforts aimed at systemwide health care savings through malpractice reform include minimizing subjective elements in determining liability, rationalizing the awards determination process, and reducing litigation costs while eliminating frivolous claims.

✦ *Determining Liability.* It is widely believed that the process of determining whether a provider is liable for damages has become excessively subjective due to an overreliance on expert witnesses with dubious qualifications and the difficulty inexperienced jurors have in distinguishing genuine negligence. This subjectivity could be reduced by establishing minimum criteria for certifying witnesses as experts in relevant areas of medicine before they are permitted to testify. Judges also could be provided with additional authority to reject a jury's finding in cases where they have inferred negligence from a mere difference in professional opinion. The process of determining negligence could be facilitated by the emerging body of research on practice guidelines.

✦ *Rationalizing the Awards Determination Process.* Another approach is to limit awards, particularly in the case of punitive damages. About twenty-five states have imposed limits on malpractice awards, which are believed to have reduced malpractice claims costs in these states by as much as 25 percent.[20] Moreover, states can require periodic payments instead

of lifetime awards, settlements provided during a plaintiff's lifetime ending upon death, and reduced payments when other sources of funding are found (e.g., disability payments or workers' compensation). They also can establish systems in which informed judges or arbitrators determine awards rather than juries.

It also has been proposed that punitive damages be awarded only in cases where there is evidence of grave dereliction of professional responsibility or reckless departure from accepted standards of practice. Mere negligence would not be a basis for punitive damages. Moreover, when punitive damages are awarded they would go to the state, not the plaintiff. This retains for the plaintiff those awards compensating the individual for personal loss, while reserving punitive judgments as a fine for gross infractions of accepted medical practice.

✦ *Reducing Litigation Costs.* A prime objective of malpractice reform is to reduce the cost of litigation without encouraging frivolous claims. Under the existing system, the high cost of the lengthy litigation process is perhaps the only deterrent to filing an unsubstantiated claim. Any effort to streamline the malpractice process must therefore be coupled with a program to prevent frivolous filings.

Some states are exploring methods to accelerate the claims process through arbitration, mediation, and summary jury trials. Neutral evaluation has been suggested as a means of eliminating frivolous claims early in the process. The American Medical Association also has proposed reducing the reliance on the jury system through arbitration by triers of fact with the necessary expertise to evaluate claims. These administrative changes could

Missouri took advantage of its legal expense fund—a self-insurance fund provided by the state to cover liabilities of state employees—as a way to expand access to obstetrical care. It now permits coverage of private physicians providing prenatal, delivery, or child care services under contract with a local health department. The program has resulted in two incentives for providers to continue to provide obstetrical care. First, the fund eliminates a provider's liability when serving these special populations. Second, the program has created an atmosphere in which malpractice insurance carriers are inclined to reduce rates. One of the major carriers in the state has reduced premiums for physicians participating in the fund by $10,000 to $15,000 a year. Additional carriers have contacted the state to learn more about the fund.

reduce litigation costs by reducing the number of unsubstantiated filings. At the same time, they could accelerate settlements for those plaintiffs with legitimate claims.

The contingency fee structure of malpractice litigation also has come under scrutiny. While the system improves access to the courts for plaintiffs with modest means, some believe it leads to a "get rich quick" mentality and litigation of unwarranted claims. Contingency fees could be regulated through limits on fees or court review of fees on a case-by-case basis.

Potential Savings from Malpractice Reform. The impact of these various liability reform approaches on systemwide health care costs currently is uncertain. Proponents of reform argue that the potential savings are sizable because of its potential to decrease liability insurance costs, decrease the excessive use of medical procedures, and ameliorate physician shortages in important practice areas. Others assert that lower malpractice insurance costs are unlikely to result in significant reductions in provider charges. Moreover, an outstanding question is how much practitioners will actually reduce defensive medicine practices in response to restricted malpractice claims, given that the risk of legal action will continue to exist. Some observers thus have argued that malpractice reform as a cost containment strategy should be considered in combination with other approaches, especially managed care strategies aimed at excess utilization.

WILL INCREMENTAL COST CONTROL STRATEGIES WORK?

Containing the growth in state health spending will require a combination of assertive management of care provided under state

health programs, and programs designed to reduce systemwide increases in health care costs. Within the context of the existing health care system, utilization controls and aggressive negotiation of provider discounts are the best means available for containing health care costs in state programs. In fact, as long as other employers are negotiating favorable discounts, the state must aggressively pursue comparable discounts to prevent providers from shifting costs to the state.

Although the experiences of individual states differ, there is evidence that states can slow the growth in statewide health spending through rate regulation and control of capital and technology, provided the process can be depoliticized and insulated from special interests. Increased participation in the regulatory process by all payors for care, particularly private industry, can enhance cost-conscious decisionmaking in the regulatory process. Expanded use of managed care and malpractice reform together could substantially reduce unnecessary care, and ensure that high-cost technologies are used in an appropriate and cost-effective manner. Empirical analysis indicates that a reduction in the rate of increase in health spending of 1 percent per year would reduce health care spending by nearly 9 percent below projected levels in 2000 (see Figure 10).

Although incremental cost containment strategies hold great promise, they also have important limitations. Most of the available approaches are aimed at a one-time reduction in health care costs, and have much less capacity to control the underlying upward pressure on costs created by advancing medical technologies. While states may be able to use these incremental approaches to limit costs for a given year or a given series of years, their longer term impact will be limited. For this reason consideration also should be given to more fundamental health system reforms. In the long run, growth in health care spending cannot be controlled until it is rationalized through systemic health care reform that balances the issues of cost, access, and quality.

ENDNOTES

1. Lewin/ICF estimate using the Health Benefit Simulation Model; and Health Care Financing Administration estimate, May 1991.

2. Lewin/ICF, *The Health Care Financing System and the Uninsured* (Washington, D.C.: Lewin/ICF, April 4, 1990).

3. Mark Chassin, Presentation to the Florida Task Force on Government Financed Health Care, September 1990.

4. Martin E. Segal Company, "Rise in State Employee Health Plan Costs Moderates: Survey of State Employee Health Benefit Plans, Summary of Findings" (New York, N.Y.: Martin E. Segal Company, 1990).

5. American Hospital Association, Special Committee on Care for the Indigent, *Cost and Comparison: Recommendations for Avoiding a Crisis in Care for the Medically Indigent* (Chicago, Ill.: American Hospital Association, 1986).

6. Jill D. Foley, *Uninsured in the United States: The Nonelderly Population without Health Insurance* (Washington, D.C.: Employee Benefit Research Institute, 1991), p. 45.

7. Lewin/ICF, 1990.

8. R.R. Bovbjerg and C.F. Koller, "State Health Insurance Pools: Current Performance, Future Prospects," *Inquiry*, vol. 23 (summer 1986).

9. Milton Roemer and Max Shain, *Hospital Utilization Under Insurance* (Chicago, Ill.: American Hospital Association, 1959).

10. Paul B. Ginsberg and Daniel M. Koretz, "Bed Availability and Hospital Utilization: Estimates of the Roemer Effect," *HCFA Review*, fall 1983.

11. Frank A. Sloan and Bruce Steinwald, "Effects of Regulation on Hospital Costs and Input Use," *Journal of Law and Economics*, April 1980.

12. John W. Mayo and Deborah A. McFarland, "Regulation, Market Structure, and Hospital Costs," *Southern Economic Journal*, 55 (January 1989).

13. Ann Lawthers-Higgins, Cynthia Taft, and Jane Hodgman, "The Impact of Certificate of Need on CAT Scanning in Massachusetts," *Health Care Management Review*, summer 1984.

14. Clark C. Havighurst and Robert S. McDonough, "The Lithotripsy Game in North Carolina: A New Technology Under Regulation and Deregulation," *Indiana Law Review*, vol. 19, no. 4 (1986).

15. C.J. Schramm, S.C. Renn, and B. Biles, "New Perspectives on State Rate Setting," *Health Affairs*, fall 1986.

16. Merton D. Finkler, "State Rate Setting Revisited," *Health Affairs*, vol. 6, no. 4 (winter 1987).

17. F.A. Sloan and W.B. Schwartz, "More Doctors: What Will They Cost?" *Journal of the American Medical Association*, 1983.

18. Sara Rosenbaum and Dana Hughes, "Appendix C: The Medical Malpractice Crisis and Poor Women," in *Prenatal Care: Reaching Mothers, Reaching Infants* (Washington, D.C.: National Academy Press, 1988).

19. National Leadership Commission on Health Care, *For the Health of a Nation: A Shared Responsibility* (Ann Arbor, Mich.: Health Administration Press, 1989).

20. F.A. Sloan, D.M. Mergenhagen, and R.R. Bovbjerg, "Effects of Tort Reforms on the Value of Closed Medical Malpractice Claims: A Microanalysis," *Journal of Health Politics, Policy and Law*, winter 1989.

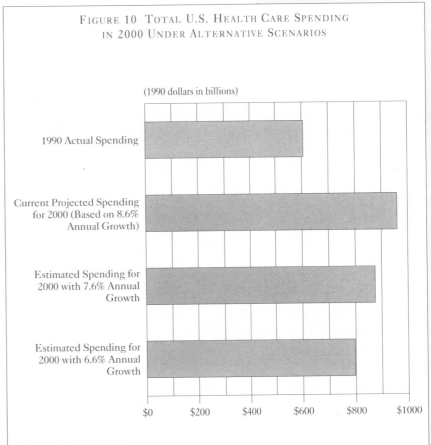

FIGURE 10 TOTAL U.S. HEALTH CARE SPENDING IN 2000 UNDER ALTERNATIVE SCENARIOS

(1990 dollars in billions)

1990 Actual Spending

Current Projected Spending for 2000 (Based on 8.6% Annual Growth)

Estimated Spending for 2000 with 7.6% Annual Growth

Estimated Spending for 2000 with 6.6% Annual Growth

$0 $200 $400 $600 $800 $1000

Source: Lewin/ICF, 1991.

Undertaking Structural Change

SUMMARY The high cost of health care is having a direct and increasing impact on every individual and business in the United States. The failure to control costs will cause the standard of living of Americans to continue to erode. While the underlying reasons for the cost explosion are complex, it is clear that health care is a unique "good" and that the industry cannot be characterized as a well-functioning market. Given these factors, state policymakers have only two choices: to move toward a more market-oriented approach, or to involve government in the allocation of health care resources.

Numerous strategies can be implemented to make the market more competitive, from providing more price and medical outcome information to initiating insurance reform. For those who believe that government intervention would be more effective in holding down costs, the all-payor model and the single-payor model are two alternatives.

All of the models have different trade-offs in terms of cost control, access, and quality, and these need to be analyzed carefully. Further, they all represent bold approaches that are oriented toward making major changes in how health care is delivered and financed. All would require substantial leadership and a sustained commitment by the Governor. Ultimately, the decision must be a political one—that is, what kind of health care system will the electorate support?

WHAT ARE THE IMPLICATIONS OF THE HIGH COST OF HEALTH CARE?

While the lack of access to health care is a national concern, its impact is limited to certain populations. The high cost of health care, on the other hand, has a direct and increasing impact on every individual and business in the United States. Furthermore, the perceived risk of becoming ill and not having the financial means to pay for care is a major worry to every American.

The major cost concerns include the following:

✦ In 1989 a worker paid at the national average hourly wage needed to work 4.8 weeks to cover household health care costs, compared with 3.3 weeks in 1980 (see Figure 11). Individuals and families spent $216 billion out of pocket for health care in 1989, an increase of 9.9 percent over the previous year.[1] This growth in health care spending reduces the money available for people to purchase other critical goods and services, such as food, housing, and transportation.

✦ From the standpoint of American business, health care costs have soared during the last twenty-five years. For example, health care costs paid by business rose from 2 percent to 7 percent of total compensation between 1965 and 1989, and from 14 percent to about 100 percent of corporate after-tax profits during the same period.[2] Health care costs are part of the cost of doing business and thus are included in the price of final products. This often puts U.S. corporations at a competitive disadvantage relative to many other industrialized countries, particularly those that have universal health care funded through income taxes. In addition to the competitive problems it causes, firms also hold down wage increases since health care costs are a significant component of total employee compensation. Health care costs often are considered the major uncontrollable cost for many firms.

✦ The fact that health care spending totals more than $600 billion and has been inflating at more than 10 percent per year also makes it a macroeconomic concern.[3] The size and rate of increase are contributing to a higher rate of general inflation in the U.S. economy. This makes it difficult for monetary and fiscal policies to stabilize the economy in the rapidly changing international marketplace.

All of these factors affect the standard of living for all Americans. The nation's failure to enact effective cost control strategies means that the real wages of U.S. citizens will continue to erode as health care cost inflation continues to accelerate.

WHAT IS THE NATURE OF THE HEALTH CARE MARKET?

Health care in the United States cannot be characterized as a well-functioning market in which consumers operate within their budget constraints to maximize the value of the services they buy, and in which prices emerge from the balance of supply and demand. Despite efforts in recent years to make the health care market more disciplined, most would argue that these changes have achieved limited success and that there still is little price competition in this industry. There are few incentives in the current system for most providers to offer, or for consumers to buy, more cost-effective products.

The fee-for-service system provides an incentive for doctors to provide more, not less, care. Once insured, particularly if a substantial amount is paid by an employer, consumers do not look at the cost of service as an important variable in their health care decisions. Essentially, physicians are making health care decisions. The subsidies built into the tax laws for employer-paid health insurance provide incentives to overinsure. Moreover, there is a cultural tendency in this nation to accept new technology, even if it is not cost-effective. This is an industry where many of the incentives cause people with insurance to overconsume health care, and for insurance companies to compete by shifting financial risk.

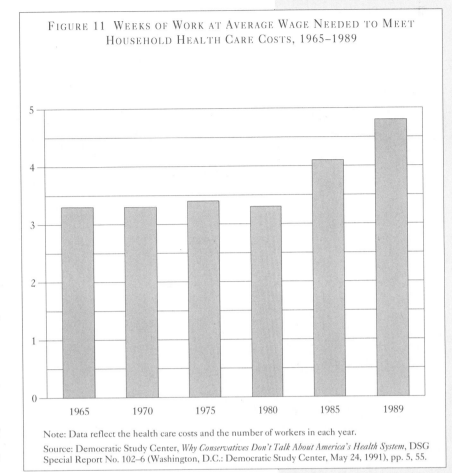

FIGURE 11 WEEKS OF WORK AT AVERAGE WAGE NEEDED TO MEET HOUSEHOLD HEALTH CARE COSTS, 1965–1989

Note: Data reflect the health care costs and the number of workers in each year.

Source: Democratic Study Center, *Why Conservatives Don't Talk About America's Health System*, DSG Special Report No. 102–6 (Washington, D.C.: Democratic Study Center, May 24, 1991), pp. 5, 55.

The market for health care therefore departs from the competitive market model in several major ways:

✦ The dynamics of the relationships among consumers, providers, and purchasers, coupled with the accelerating rate of technological change, have resulted in most consumers delegating their decisionmaking to providers. Consumers are averting the risk associated with making their own decisions.

✦ The emergence of third-party payors (e.g., insurance companies and employer-paid insurance) has insulated consumers from making cost-effective decisions.

✦ Both the uncertainty of illness and the tax subsidy to employer-paid health insurance have encouraged consumers to demand a higher quantity of service than is economically prudent.

✦ The existence of multiple payors dilutes the incentives for providers to hold down costs. Each hospital and doctor receives payments from numerous sources, including patients, insurers, HMOs, and Medicaid and Medicare. The true cost of services is seldom known, and so there is little incentive to make cost-effective decisions.

As a result of these factors, the cost or price of health care is seldom a major input into health care decisions. Essentially, it is the perception of quality—often decided by the provider—that is the critical decisionmaking variable. This does not contribute to an effective market that provides high quality, low-cost services.

WHAT ARE THE OPTIONS?
MARKET VERSUS PUBLIC ALLOCATION

Given that the current incentives in the marketplace are not working to hold down health care costs, what are the options for policymakers? One option is to move closer to a market approach and to regulate the marketplace only where there are major market failures. A second option is to involve government in decisions about the allocation of health care resources.

These proposals go beyond incremental approaches by recommending that the entire health care financing system in a state be restructured. The proposals would modify the current system of multiple, independent payors with either a system driven by competitive market forces in which hospitals, nursing homes, doctors, and other health care providers bid for customers or groups of customers by offering lower prices; or a uniform payment system that centralizes payments to such health care providers. Both proposals would force providers to reduce costs in order to remain profitable.

Any of the proposals described here could substantially reduce the growth of health expenditures in a state. It is likely that it will be difficult to make the transition to these models, but they may offer the only real opportunities for sustained cost control.

Governors need to be aware that in considering these strategies, they are plunging into a contentious debate between two schools of thought about how to achieve major health care cost containment. Looking at the same facts, cost figures, and behavior in the current health care system, each school reaches different conclusions about the shape of reform needed.

The first school of thought advocates the adoption of competitive market reforms to reduce health spending. The approach and reasoning of this group is very similar to that of proponents of deregulation and increased competitive activity for the airline, trucking, banking, and long-distance telephone industries. With the right incentives for individual consumers and the proper procompetitive regulatory structures, there will be a sharp rise in the number of new health organizations (involving various combinations of hospitals, medical groups, and insurers) competing for enrollees based on the lowest prices and most effective use of health resources.

The second school includes those who favor enactment of an all-payor (or even single-payor) system and a prospectively established yearly budget or financial limit on health services expenditures and health-related capital expenditures within a state. Health care decisions and priority setting would take place within the context of an agreed-upon spending limit on almost all private and public health expenditures. Growth in the spending limit would be tied to some reasonable projected growth rate, such as growth in the state economy.

Governors will have to decide their own preferences based on prior deregulation efforts, the efficacy of earlier programs of state utility regulation, and whether the experience of foreign health care systems is applicable to the United States or their own state. Additionally, the politics of the state, past interactions with the state legislature, the goals of the state in containing costs and improving access to care, and the likelihood of getting federal flexibility (e.g., waivers) should be considered.

In practice, Governors do not have to choose policies exclusively from either of the two schools of thought. They are described as separate approaches only for ease of presentation. It is recognized that various options within the models could be included in a single reform initiative. However, to have a broad impact one needs to understand the differences in emphasis and focus between the two alternatives for cost containment. Only then can specific state proposals for health care reform be assessed.

While the effectiveness of the two strategies in controlling costs is critical, there are important trade-offs. Regardless of the options that are pursued, Governors must consider their potential impact not only on cost, but also on access and quality of care. For example, it is likely that the public allocation model would bring costs down faster and perhaps even further than the competitive approach. However, it is likely that consumers would have to give up some freedom of choice (e.g., when and where they can schedule surgery). Moreover, the public allocation model could have a negative impact on the rate of technology dissemination and even development. This could translate into a decline in quality. In contrast, the competitive model may be less effective in controlling costs. The removal of barriers to providers entering the market may result in an overall decline in the quality of care.

The Market Model

In theory, the market model is a simple concept. It assumes that all buyers and sellers have ample knowledge regarding the prices, quality, and quantity of output. There should be a sufficient number of buyers and sellers so that none has a significant influence over the price or quantity of any given service. Also, there should be no major impediments or restrictions on the marketplace. Most important, services demanded by consumers must be available by providers at minimum cost. With lower costs and prices, more consumers would be able to afford to purchase health care, thus increasing access. While such a model never truly exists in the real world, there are a number of policies a state could implement to make health care more market-oriented.

This model assumes that competition will be enhanced and costs will be reduced through increased information and the reduction of market imperfections. Only where there are major market failures would a government entity regulate or enter the market. This model could be adjusted toward more managed competition, though such a strategy would liken cost containment to the incremental changes outlined in the previous chapter.

Under the market model, health care costs would be lowered when consumers are given sufficient incentives to use lower cost health delivery systems and insurance plans. Essentially, the view is that health care costs will be lower in the future if the priorities for health and medicine are set by individual consumers through their choice of health plans, including benefits and the level of services. Moving toward a more market-oriented strategy would require the following state actions.

Enhance Information. For the market model to work effectively, it is critical that all purchasers have ample information to make rational decisions. Specifically, prices for the entire continuum of health services must be readily available, including prices for insurance packages, office visits, surgical procedures, and hospital stays. Moreover, it is important to have medical outcome information by type of service and provider. States

can play an important role in ensuring that the information is available and that purchasers and consumers are educated about how to use the information to make cost-effective decisions. A state could collect and publish the information directly or encourage other groups to provide it.

Change the Tax Status of Health Benefits. A critical component of a competitive strategy is for state government to encourage employers to establish maximum limits on their contributions to their employees' premiums. Whatever level of premium sharing each employer chooses, it would be applied as a percentage of the lowest cost health insurance plan available in the employee's geographic area. The employee still has a choice of plans, but the amount the employee pays is larger for the more expensive plans. This would force employees to choose the most cost-effective package of services or to pay more for enhanced services. Currently, many employers contribute more for more expensive programs, making out-of-pocket costs for employees virtually the same for all plans.

To change the level of premium sharing, a state could limit employers' corporate tax deduction for contributions to their employees' insurance premiums to a certain percentage. States also could cap employees' health benefit tax deduction for state income taxes. With a change in the tax status of health benefits, employers would be less likely to provide benefits beyond the level of the tax benefit, and employees would be more likely to choose the health care options that are least expensive.

Eliminate Mandates on Insurance Benefits. A significant number of states mandate that insurance policies include certain benefits, such as in vitro fertilization and chiropractic care. While the additional costs associated with these mandates are relatively small (3 percent to 12 percent), they do increase costs and reduce the ability of health care plans to compete in terms of the type of coverage they provide.

Reduce Barriers to Entry for Providers. Most states have laws that restrict the development of new health plans and give existing doctors and hospitals an advantage over would-be competitors. To some degree, high health care costs can be related to the collusion between and among physicians and hospitals to restrict price-related competition. Promoting competition would require that state governments strengthen and aggressively enforce antitrust laws against health professionals and institutions that limit competition, or punish providers who discount prices or advertise. To promote the greatest efficiency in providers' costs, all barriers to entry should be removed to increase the delivery of services and drive the market toward greater efficiency and lower prices.

Similarly, certificate of need and health planning laws would need to be repealed by states since they act as mechanisms for existing providers to restrict entry into the market and thus stifle competition. States pursuing these policies would need to change their corporate medical practice laws to allow hospitals and physicians to collaborate for the joint sale of medical and hospital services, and reduce provider certification requirements to the minimum needed for public safety. Less restrictive medical licensure laws would need to be enacted to permit an expanded role for, and more widespread use of, less costly health

personnel such as nurse-midwives and physician assistants. Finally, state governments would not intervene to bail out failing hospitals, insurers, or HMOs unless they were the sole source of health care in an area.

Encourage Small Employer Buyer Groups. Many employers are not large enough to exercise sufficient market power in negotiating with health care providers who will seriously concern themselves with cost containment. This is an example of a real market failure where providers are in a position to take advantage of purchasers. One approach to promoting a more efficient system would be to establish state-sponsored consortiums of small employers that would solicit bids from insurers or health maintenance organizations that want to provide complete coverage at a competitive price. An added benefit of the consortium approach would be to lower the high administrative costs currently associated with small business insurance plans.

This option would require enabling legislation similar to that for producer cooperatives that currently exist for goods such as for milk and cranberries. The difference is that the state-sponsored small employer consortium would be for purchasers rather than providers. Not unlike large-scale defense contracting, the employers in these consortiums would specify in advance the mix and type of insurers, hospital services, emergency coverage, and medical specialty services needed. Based on a price bid and an independent assessment of the quality of the physicians and hospitals, the employers would choose one or more health care plans as the exclusive provider of health care services for their employees in each geographic area of the state.

Implement Insurance Reforms. Current insurance practice is to compete by shifting the risk of large potential medical costs instead of lowering costs. As a result, many businesses with high-risk employees either pay very high rates or are not able to obtain coverage. Again, this is an example of a major market failure. A competitive cost containment approach would require state government to eliminate adverse selection in the sale of health insurance policies so that price competition is based on the cost of the medical care provided rather than the health risk of employees. Many states have dealt with this problem in the automobile insurance market by limiting the number of factors that can be used in setting prices for policies, and by requiring an open enrollment period each year during which employers may purchase an insurance plan. Other reforms would require insurance policies to be community-rated (or standard risk-rated) so that firms would pay the same price for coverage, regardless of the age, sex, or health status of their employees.

Eliminate Hidden Subsidies. States also would need to eliminate hidden subsidies in health insurance reimbursement policies that make some plans less cost-competitive. Individual insurers in the state would need to be relieved of the subsidy they currently pay for uncompensated charity care in order to compete with payors that do not contribute to this subsidy. The uncompensated charity care subsidy would be replaced by direct payments by state government either through a public insurance program or a voucher program similar to Food Stamps.

Establish a Public Agency to Manage Competition. States would need to designate a lead agency to oversee the operation of the various components of this market approach, similar to the Civil Aeronautics Board for the airline industry. This agency would monitor the small employers' group bidding and ensure that each business held an annual open enrollment with wide choice. It would be responsible for facilitating consumer participation by requiring that standard cost and quality information is released to the public, press, and employers on a routine basis. For example, it would publish the mortality rates for bypass surgery at each hospital in the state performing such surgeries. Employees could then select their health plan with adequate knowledge of the impact of their decisions on the quality and cost of care they would receive from the providers participating in each plan. The agency also would enforce antitrust laws. Finally, the agency would have an advisory board composed of representatives of business, labor, government, providers, insurers, and consumers.

Make Consumers Conscious of Health Care Costs. Many would argue that the decline in the share of health service costs paid by individual consumers has been a major cause of the rapid increase in spending for health services during the past twenty-five years. For example, studies by the RAND Corporation during the late 1970s and early 1980s found that "spending per person was 45 percent higher in a plan that required no cost sharing compared with a plan that required 95 percent cost sharing up to an annual maximum of $1,000."[4] States could encourage employers to establish deductibles and copayments to force consumers to make more cost-effective health care utilization decisions. Of course, increased cost sharing would have a disproportionate impact on low- and middle-income people.

The Public Allocation Model

Unlike the market-driven model, the public allocation model calls for greater intervention on the part of state government. Within this model, two alternatives are possible: an all-payor model that would cause only minor dislocations to the current health care industry, and a single-payor model that would offer the potential for greater cost savings, but at the risk of more short-run dislocation to the industry.

Those who advocate a public allocation model argue that health care should not be left to the vagaries of a competitive market. This is because individuals do not have adequate independent knowledge to make decisions about what is medically needed and what is appropriate care. Unlike most other types of consumer goods, patients are totally dependent on someone else (i.e., their doctor) to make health care decisions on their behalf. As a result, the costs of health care are principally determined by the behavior of the service providers, and therefore public policy should focus on altering their financial behavior. Further, advocates of this approach argue that governmental intervention often is required to resolve conflicts between the broad societal goal of improving the health of all citizens and the goal of providers to provide care while enhancing their own financial viability. Moreover, protection of the public interest requires certain restrictions that limit the possibility of marketplace competition, including limits on professional licensure and practice, accreditation, medical specialty certification, and prescription authority. In many cases, hospitals and other health care facilities are essential institutions to their communities, and thus decisions about whether they should expand, reduce their capacity, or close must be public

decisions and not a result of marketplace forces alone. Finally, some believe there are substantial economies of scale to be achieved through a single purchaser, and thus significant savings are possible if government makes the allocation decisions.

The All-Payor Model. One approach for a state is to implement an all-payor model. An all-payor system centralizes health care payment decisions in a single quasi-public agency that negotiates health care prices or payments between providers and purchasers of care.

Implementation of an all-payor model would proceed sequentially as follows:

✦ Creation of a quasi-public agency to implement the system;

✦ Development of a common billing system;

✦ Negotiation of fees for all providers;

✦ Negotiation of a ceiling for health services expenditures; and

✦ Negotiation of a ceiling for capital expenditures for health care.

While the potential for cost reduction will increase as a state proceeds through this sequence of steps, so do the probabilities for political conflict. Therefore, a state may wish to phase in the steps to allow sufficient time to evaluate their impact.

The major advantage of an all-payor system is that it gives purchasers leverage in negotiating with providers in order to control the growth in health spending. Other advantages of this system are:

✦ It pays providers uniform rates, reducing their motivation to shift costs among payors.

✦ It achieves some economies of scale that reduce administrative costs.

✦ It improves access to care because payment rates are equalized among purchasers, thus

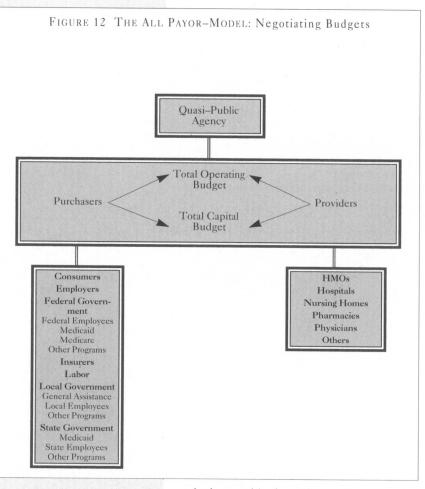

FIGURE 12 THE ALL PAYOR–MODEL: Negotiating Budgets

could be saved nationally through common billing forms and procedures.[5] The state could take the initiative in developing and implementing such a system.

✦ *Negotiate Fees for All Providers.* Third, the state would give the agency the authority to negotiate fees for all providers. All purchasers, including consumers, would pay the negotiated rate for health services. While such an approach could be limited to hospitals, it would be more effective in reducing total health care costs if it applied equally to nursing homes, prescription drugs, and physicians. Maryland, Massachusetts, New Jersey, and New York had all-payor systems for hospitals in place for a number of years. However, only Maryland continues to have a system that establishes both a reimbursement methodology and actual rates paid to hospitals. Evaluations of these systems found that they reduced the rate of increase in health care costs. However, restricting the scope of rate setting to a single type of service (e.g., inpatient hospital care) may lead to increases in the use of other types of services.

✦ *Negotiate a Ceiling for Health Services Expenditures.* To prevent increases in the use of other types of services, the agency would want to negotiate a ceiling or so-called global operating budget for health services expenditures. The goal of a global health care budget could be to bring the rate of growth in health care costs down close to the general inflation rate. Actual budget growth, however, could reflect not only inflation, but also adjustments for the aging of the population and large changes in utilization due to epidemics and the introduction of important new technologies.

reducing provider incentives to deny care due to differential reimbursement.

✦ *Create a Quasi-Public Agency to Implement the System.* The state could create a quasi-public agency composed of representatives from both providers and purchasers. It is important that the agency be at least quasi-public so it can negotiate on behalf all payors without risk of antitrust violation.

✦ *Develop a Common Billing System.* Next, a common billing system would be developed for all providers that balances purchasers' needs for information and providers' interests in minimizing barriers to reimbursement. One study has indicated that more than $30 billion in hospital and physician administrative costs

Establishing a global operating budget would occur under the auspices of the quasi-public agency and would take place in two stages. (The first stage is shown in Figure 12.) First, purchasers and providers would meet independently. The group of purchasers (business and labor groups, federal, state, and local governments, insurance companies, and representatives of the self-employed) would agree on their target expenditure based on the resources they contribute to the system, including total dollars and total beneficiaries. The group of providers (hospitals, nursing homes, physician groups, health maintenance organizations, and pharmaceutical representatives) would engage in similar discussions based on the kinds and number of services they contribute. Second, provider and purchaser representatives would meet under the authority of the quasi-public agency and negotiate, much like is done within the automobile industry between manufacturers and the United Auto Workers. These discussions would take place simultaneously since the process would have to be interactive. The agency's role in the negotiation process could take several forms, including gathering data and information to set the context for negotiations, providing protection from antitrust, and enforcing the results of the negotiations.

Providers who refuse to participate could be paid a maximum of the previous year's rate, adjusted for changes in utilization. Purchasers who refuse to participate would not gain the negotiated rate advantage. The ultimate objective is to agree on a total for health services expenditures.

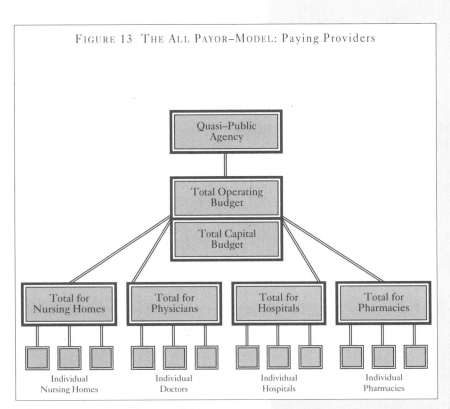

FIGURE 13 THE ALL PAYOR–MODEL: Paying Providers

Payments to providers would be accomplished as shown in Figure 13. In the first year the proportion going to each provider group could be roughly what it is now, but over time there would be a reallocation depending on utilization. If any provider overran its budget in a year, that amount would be reduced from the next year's allocation. This control would likely cause providers to set up their own utilization review boards to prevent such overruns. Similarly, each purchaser group would contribute roughly what it contributes now, but over time there would be a reallocation depending on changes in their relative market share.

Setting a budget is crucial to the success of all-payor system. Without it, a state can control only fees, not utilization. The budget allocation process requires providers to pay attention not only to their fees, but also to the number of services they deliver.

✦ *Negotiate a Ceiling for Capital Expenditures for Health Care.* Next, the state would control capital expenditures by both existing and new facilities and for technology through a capital budget and approval process. (This step could be done prior to negotiating a global operating budget for health services expenditures.) Revenue for the capital budget could be generated from a designated capital charge on all provider billings or from funds contributed by all payors. The capital budget could be separated into two components: one designated for facility construction and improvement, and one for the introduction and dissemination of technology. The capital budgets would be distributed through negotiations within the quasi-public agency.

The model for this type of capital control is found in most states in the public higher education system, which makes all capital apportionment decisions centrally and then allocates the funds among state colleges and universities. Unlike health care providers, state colleges and universities are not allowed to borrow whatever they need without receiving approval through the state budgetary process that determines how much expansion the state can afford. If a state were to change its payment system as outlined here, capital controls would become critical to controlling overall health care inflation, and denying some requests would likely be necessary to stay within the negotiated ceiling.

The Single-Payor Model. While implementation of an all-payor system clearly would provide cost savings, additional efficiencies could be attained by moving to a single-payor or single-source financing system. Such a system would require substantial changes in the financing, production, and delivery of health services. While an example of a single-payor system does not exist in the United States, several models are in use in Canada and Europe. The essential characteristics of this approach—whether one adopts a tax-based financing system (as in Canada, Great Britain, or the Nordic countries) or a social insurance model (as in Germany or the Netherlands)—is that all health care funds pass through a single publicly controlled (in the tax-based systems) or publicly accountable (in the social insurance systems) financing mechanism.

A tax-based approach relies on general revenue, which can be raised at the national, regional, or local level. Typically these revenues are raised through personal income taxes, with each level setting its own rates. The second type of single-source financing system involves fixed social insurance contributions, typically split between employers and employees. These contributions are assessed on a community basis, with employees paying a fixed percentage of their income regardless of whether they have dependents or health-related conditions. Employers contribute through a payroll tax.

An important distinction between the two types of single-source systems concerns the day-to-day administration of the financing system. In a tax-based system, administration generally is handled by an agency of the national, regional, or municipal government. This agency is directly politically accountable for its decisions, an advantage or disadvantage depending on one's perspective. In a social insurance-based system, administrative matters typically are handled by quasi-independent bodies that are governed by employer and employee representatives.

In tax-based and social insurance models alike, single-source financing is essential not only to controlling aggregate spending levels, but also to steering provider policy on the quality and composition of services. These two policy objectives are pursued in tax-based systems through a combination of ownership of hospitals and bilateral negotiations with hospitals and physicians. Thus, the national, regional, or municipal government body that controls and/or influences the revenue flow serves as a countervailing power to resource demands from hospitals and physicians.

In social insurance-based systems, negotiations typically do not involve governmental bodies. Rather, an association of the national or regional social insurance funds negotiates with a parallel association of physicians. These negotiations occur regardless of whether the physicians are private entrepreneurs (private practitioners in Canada, Denmark, Germany, Great Britain, and the Netherlands) or salaried civil servants at the regional or municipal level. Hospital negotiations take place only where hospitals are not owned and operated by the government authority that controls financing. For example, each Canadian provincial government and the hospitals negotiate the size of prospective global budgets. In social insurance-based systems, the negotiations follow the same pattern as for physicians, occurring between the national or regional association of sick funds and individual hospitals.

At present, major reform processes are underway in nearly every European health system. This does not indicate that there is no system that works well, but rather that important aspects of system design are time-sensitive. What may be a distinct advantage at one point in the development of a health system may become a distinct disadvantage ten years later. Thus, one key lesson from the experience of single-source financing systems is that they must be seen as dynamic structures, and must be capable of evolving as conditions change.

Viewed from the perspective of state capitols in the United States, public allocation financing models have clear and apparent advantages over the present system:

◆ They would provide a stable funding base for the provision of health services.

◆ They would allow state government to cap health-related expenditures.

◆ They would be simple and less expensive to administer. They are simple in that all purchasers would know in advance how much they would spend on health care and providers would know how much they would receive. Administrative paperwork for purchasers and providers for reimbursement and payment would be reduced considerably.

◆ With control over a single financing mechanism, states could more readily implement policy objectives such as the provision of more preventive and primary care.

◆ States could implement a system using a mix of provider reimbursement models (capitation, salary, and/or fee-for-service).

◆ The entire bilateral negotiation strategy can be implemented at the state level. States are regional in the same sense as provinces in Canada or counties in Sweden. If the appropriate waivers could be obtained from the federal Health Care Financing Administration, a state could require that all payments be channeled through a statewide negotiation process built on associations of hospitals and of physicians.

This optimistic picture of the advantages of the public allocation model for states must be tempered with an assessment of the disadvantages that could accompany the introduction of such a system by one or more state governments:

✦ State government would have to generate the political will to act boldly in the face of probable intense lobbying and advertising from sectors within the health care industry.

✦ State government would need to demonstrate to its citizens that it is competent to assume the major responsibilities that a publicly controlled or publicly accountable financing system entails.

✦ Individual states would run the risk of triggering two perverse migrations: one of small industry out of the state (to avoid paying any health insurance costs at all), the other of chronically ill and/or disabled persons into the state (to gain access to a universal system).

✦ There is no guarantee that the model would not suffer from at least some measure of provider influence.

✦ There would be a danger of administrative rigidity. If public control were not balanced by a sufficient degree of local flexibility, the ability of the overall system to respond to changes in technology could be reduced.

✦ Capping total health care spending may require longer waits for certain services, which could increase consumer dissatisfaction with the model.

A public allocation model would not magically generate new health care revenues for existing hard-pressed delivery systems. What this approach would do is to redirect existing revenues, allowing them to be used more efficiently and effectively.

There are two major differences between the single-payor system and all-payor system.

First, because the single-payor approach is supported by a broad-based tax, it is traditionally combined with universal access. In fact, public pressures for universal access rather than cost containment may be the driving force to implement a single-payor system. Second, the single-payor system would likely have much lower administrative costs than the all-payor system. It also is true that a single-payor model could be viewed as the final step, after the all-payor model, on the continuum of cost control models.

WHAT IS NEEDED FOR STRUCTURAL REFORM?

The market model and public allocation model are both oriented toward major structural reform to significantly lower costs. Because these are bold new approaches that have not been previously implemented in the United States, it is important to consider a number of other issues in making a decision to adopt either model or any of the options within each model.

Leadership

Adopting either model would require substantial leadership by the Governor. While there is a growing consensus for major reform of the health care system, there currently is no consensus on the type of change needed. Building that consensus for major systemic reform would be difficult. Also, some of the options contained in either model would require the enactment of sweeping state legislation.

Sustained Commitment

Development, implementation, and evaluation of the adopted cost control model would require a sustained commitment. Adjustments take time, particularly in long-term investments such as the purchase of new technology and the development of new services. Moreover, it will take time to realize changes in the behavior of all parties—purchasers, consumers, and providers.

Changes in the Public Role

Whether the market model or the public allocation model is chosen, changes in the role and functions of state government can be anticipated. The Governor would need to decide how much direct control over these decisions is necessary, and how much political insulation from these issues is desirable when establishing the governance structure to implement the reform initiative. There are three alternatives. First, the Governor could create a new agency or designate an existing agency to monitor administration of the program. This arrangement is analogous to the role the Food and Drug Administration plays in overseeing the conditions for the sale and distribution of drugs, without actually owning or directing their sale. Second, the Governor could appoint an independent commission that actively oversees the workings of the health care industry. An example of such a system is the Civil Aeronautics Board, which is a government board appointed to monitor the operational policies of private airlines. Third, the Governor could designate or establish an agency to be the single payor. This is analogous to the role the Health Care Financing Administration plays for the Medicare program.

Implementation Strategy

Given that these models represent bold departures from existing approaches, a comprehensive plan is needed to implement the various components in an appropriate sequence. Also, it may be important to phase in the changes. This would allow sufficient opportunity to evaluate the impact of each of the steps and, if necessary, to modify the course.

Federal Policy Changes

As the various cost containment strategies are developed at the state level, it is important that they be fully integrated with federal policy. This means that states will need to be continually aware of the opportunities or barriers that federal policy changes could pose for their structural reform efforts. Moreover, some federal policy changes may be necessary, for example, to get Medicare and Medicaid to participate in global budgeting negotiations.

WHAT DOES THIS MEAN FOR GOVERNORS?

In contrast to the incremental changes described in the previous chapter, the models examined in this chapter are considered to be major structural reforms. As such, they assume that the current incentives and behavioral responses in the health care market will not lead to sustained cost control. The difficulty is that there is very little empirical evidence available on which to base a decision about which route to take. Ultimately, the decision must be a political one—that is, what kind of health care system will the electorate support?

ENDNOTES

1. Katharine R. Levit and Cathy A. Cowan, "The Burden of Health Care Costs: Business, Households, and Governments," *Health Care Financing Review*, vol. 12, no. 2 (winter 1990), p. 129.

2. Levit, p. 134.

3. Helen C. Lazenby and Suzanne W. Letsch, "National Health Expenditures, 1989," *Health Care Financing Review*, vol. 12, no. 2 (winter 1990), p. 1.

4. Congressional Budget Office, *Rising Health Care Costs: Causes, Implications, and Strategies* (Washington, D.C.: U.S. Government Printing Office, April 1991), p. 34.

5. U.S. General Accounting Office, *Canadian Health Insurance: Lessons for the United States* (Washington, D.C.: U.S. General Accounting Office, June 1991), p. 7.

The Opportunity

SUMMARY The current U.S. health care system does not serve the best interests of anyone. Costs—both public and private—are out of control. And despite the $700 billion the nation spends on health care each year, many Americans are deprived of access to needed services.

Some fear that changing the current system will make things worse. In fact, a more efficient system may be able to provide universal access without added costs. Reform should not be feared; indeed, the challenges represent an exciting opportunity for all those in the system.

States considering making fundamental, structural changes to their health care system can follow one of three approaches, each of which reflects a different allocation of responsibility between the public and private sectors. They can:

✦ Create a single private system using public funds as a source of subsidies and reinsurance;

✦ Move away from the current employer-based system; or

✦ Publicly finance basic health care and use private insurance for catastrophic coverage.

WHAT PREMISES ARE KEY TO SUCCESS?

A variety of policy options are available to Governors to achieve the dual goals of universal access and cost containment. The choices range from minor incremental changes to achieve cost savings, to a major restructuring of the organization and financing of health care. The direction a Governor ultimately takes will depend on his or her beliefs about the nature of health care and the way resources should be allocated. Whatever the direction, some basic premises are key to success.

✦ *There is no single solution for all states.* Depending on the state, its health care system, and its values and needs, some approaches will be more applicable than others. Some states might opt for solutions that rely on managing the market to achieve greater competition; others might seek a "public good" approach to the allocation of health care resources.

✦ *No single strategy will suffice.* Any significant progress toward achieving the goals of universal access and cost containment will require a combination of approaches. Whether the solution involves, for example, Medicaid expansions, employer mandates, state subsidies, or an all-payor system, each of these must be viewed as part of a more comprehensive strategy for change.

✦ *Without federal cooperation, a state will have difficulty succeeding.* The role of the federal government may be financial, including increasing Medicaid support or changing tax policy, or it may involve providing more flexibility for states to modify Medicaid and the Employee Retirement Income Security Act. Since many of the approaches initially will require testing and evaluation, federal grant support will be necessary to help plan and implement such efforts.

✦ *Strategies must encompass both goals.* Without increasing access to health insurance, the problems of cost shifting will impede efforts to contain costs. Conversely, without reducing health care costs, it may be impossible to make health insurance affordable for much of the currently uninsured population.

WHAT ARE SOME BOLDER STEPS?

Many argue that the current health care system is crumbling. They contend that the private insurance sector is neither willing nor capable of solving the problem. Opponents point to the lack of coverage for small businesses, the high rate of growth in premiums, abusive insurance practices, and a lack of good preventive and primary coverage as indications of the limits of private insurance in truly solving the American health care crisis. Many who advocate a public system claim that health care, like education, is a right and, as such, should be financed as a public good and not insured as though it is an optional luxury.

They also argue that "health insurance" is an oxymoron: one should insure against sickness, not against health. They question whether health is even an insurable event. Insurance implies a risk, but if many of the services people need are fairly predictable (e.g., preventive care), are such services most appropriately covered by insurance? Alternatively, where is the risk if insurers are trying to eliminate those who are at risk and are basing their premiums on the actual health experience of populations?

Whether one agrees with these arguments depends on one's ideology and views regarding how much change is feasible, given the nation's history and values and the entrenchment of the private sector in the health care system. Even among those who would argue for a public system, there is some disagreement as to how this actually might work.

At least in the short term, a totally public solution may be unlikely. This society tends to eschew radical solutions to problems, despite the seriousness of the crisis. Instead, the nation typically prefers incremental approaches that assume a role for both the private and public sectors in the solution.

That does not imply that the status quo must be maintained; it simply suggests that there may be other ways to combine the two sectors in order to fundamentally address the structural problems of the current system. This may be accomplished through a major reorganization of the current relationships, or achieved more incrementally over time.

Three possible approaches states might consider in making fundamental changes are described below. They are listed in order of how much restructuring of the current system would be required.

✦ Create a single private system using public funds as a source of subsidies and reinsurance;

✦ Move away from the current employer-based system; and

✦ Publicly finance basic health care and use private insurance for catastrophic coverage.

Individual states have options, with respect to both the different approaches and the degree to which they might implement such changes.

Creating a Single Private System

Under a single private system, everybody would be covered through a private insurance policy and public funds would be used to subsidize insurance for those too poor to afford such coverage without assistance. In addition, to make insurance more affordable and to ensure coverage for those deemed uninsurable, the public sector would act as a reinsurer.

In this approach, public insurance would no longer be used as a direct payor for acute care services. Every person below age sixty-five would be enrolled in a private insurance plan. The funds currently available under Medicaid would be used for both subsidies and reinsurance.

At the core of this approach is a private health insurance plan. All individuals—regardless of income, health status, or place of employment—would be eligible to enroll in one of these precertified plans. Risk would be spread across the entire plan (community-rated), rather than each enrollee or group being rated separately. However, the plan would assume only that portion of the risk up to some predetermined level for each enrollee (e.g., $25,000 per year). Any costs above that level would be covered by a public reinsurance mechanism offered by a state.

All qualifying plans would offer the same level of minimum coverage. Individuals or employees could opt for more benefits, totally at their own expense. Because of the community rating, reinsurance, restrictions on premium increases, and guaranteed renewal, the need for medical underwriting and pre-existing condition exclusions would become less of an issue. Also, since premiums would not be based on an individual employer's experience, portability for the minimum package would be ensured even if employees lost or changed their jobs.

Qualifying plans also would be required to use the same payment, billing, documentation, and coverage rules for the basic coverage. In this way, though the pluralistic system could be maintained, administrative costs would be reduced.

Support for the subsidies would be shared by the federal government and state governments. Whether this program would cost more than current total public expenditures for the nonelderly is uncertain. For many individuals, Medicaid already is the payor of high-cost care, and for those currently receiving Medicaid coverage, the cost of the subsidy to purchase private insurance may be less than the current burden on Medicaid. However, demonstrations would be necessary to determine whether, and how much, incremental costs might be associated with this approach.

More fundamental is the fact that this approach may not address many of the purported shortcomings of the private insurance industry. By leaving the basic coverage in the hands of private insurers, opponents might argue that this approach still would be insuring, rather than financing, basic care. Does this not leave the least "insurable" portion of health care in the hands of the private insurers? For example, should predictable preventive services be considered an insurable event? How does this approach stop insurance companies from "gaming" the system, creating adverse selection, and/or limiting access to high-risk individuals and industries? The answer to these questions may involve basic, philosophic attitudes toward the role, if any, of private insurance. Again, these questions might be examined further through demonstrations of this approach.

Then why pursue this approach? First, it maintains the essentially private nature of the system. Second, it may represent a more efficient use of Medicaid funds. Third, while maintaining the basic employer-based system, it eliminates many of the problems associated with that system. Last, while maintaining the private insurance industry, the approach does away with much of the fragmentation and inefficiency currently plaguing the system.

Moving Away From the Employer-Based System

The employer-based system acts as an impediment for many of the working uninsured to obtain coverage. Restructuring the system would require a change in its underlying financing.

True structural reform will require a new way to group people for insurance purposes. For example, new groupings such as those formed by unions, religious or community organizations, or school districts already have been created or are being developed.

Moving away from the employer-based system would not necessarily require the elimination of private insurance as the means of reimbursing for health care. Rather, private insurance could remain at the heart of the system; what would change is the mechanism for collecting the funds to finance the system. Plans could continue to compete on the basis of services provided to members, as well as on any supplemental benefits. Employees would pay some percentage of their income

(matched by employers) to purchase insurance. Public subsidies such as tax credits might be used to assist marginal employers, and direct government payments for premiums could be made on behalf of the unemployed. These collected funds would then be used to purchase private insurance from approved carriers and would cover an agreed-upon set of benefits. Expanded coverage would be at the option of the employer and employee, but would be purchased separately from private insurers. The progressivity of this approach is evident, but could vary depending on whether taxable maximums were used or on the share paid by the employer and employee.

In this way, many of the problems of the employer-based system can be addressed. The use of the payroll tax is, in some ways, a pure form of community rating. In other words, the premium amount paid by employers and employees is related more to their income than their health experience.

While, as in Germany, there is some variation in the payroll tax percentage based on region and industry, the risk is essentially spread across the larger population. Thus, many of the problems that cause small businesses to pay more for insurance, related both to risk and premium collection costs, can be minimized or eliminated. Insuring the total population can alleviate current problems of cost shifting caused by the uninsured and underinsured.

Medicaid and other state and local funds could be used as a part of the public subsidy. Since these funds would be leveraging private dollars, they might be sufficient to cover the added costs associated with expanded coverage. However, there is clearly a risk that added public expenditures will be needed, which would require testing if this approach were to be adopted.

Even if public costs were not increased, a more significant barrier to this approach is the added tax burden, particularly using the payroll tax. Yet, the tax burden on presently covered employers and employees would in fact be less than their current premium costs. This is so because the plan would eliminate the cost shifting present in the current system and, for small businesses, reduce the higher premiums they now are forced to pay. Depending on how the payroll tax was structured, the relative burdens of paying for health insurance might be redistributed between employers and employees. Finally, for employers and individuals who are currently uncovered, such an approach would represent an additional burden. Nevertheless, the majority of Americans would pay no more, and many even less, than their current health care costs.

At a time when there is an anti-tax sentiment in this country, the implementation of this approach remains politically problematic. This is further complicated by the fact that if a state were to implement such a program, some businesses, particularly those currently not bearing any health insurance cost, might opt to move rather than incur the added burden. These problems must be weighed against the potential savings that would accrue to many employers and employees, as well as the long-term benefits of addressing a fundamental problem within the American health care system.

A last concern about moving away from the employer-based system is that it may not address some of the problems associated with private insurance. While this plan changes the underlying mechanism for financing, it leaves the private insurance system intact. State insurance reform may address some of the problem, but the potential for "gaming" and adverse selection remain, as do the issues of whether health care is insurable or should be a public good. Again, this is a philosophical issue and would depend on how much reform accompanied this change. Before this approach could be implemented, however, demonstrations would be needed to determine the effects of altering the underlying financing, the operation of private insurance, the distribution of risk, and the potential for abuse.

Publicly Financing Basic Health Care
In the first approach, a public-private partnership was described in which private insurance would continue to offer the basic coverage, with the public sector acting as the reinsurer. This option does not address the question of whether private insurance is the appropriate mechanism to cover the more predictable aspects of health care. If one were to argue that insurance should be viewed more as a "gamble"—protecting the individual against the potential of a catastrophic event—then another alternative would be to reverse the earlier option and use private insurance to cover that risk, rather than basic services. The more basic coverage, including preventive and most primary care, might be more appropriately a public responsibility, and catastrophic care a logical role for the private sector.

For example, if basic care—possibly defined as payment for services for an individual up to $5,000 annually—were financed directly through the public sector, private insurance would then cover expenses in excess of that amount. In this way, private insurance actually would be used for more "insurable" events where the risk was greatest, and the public sector would ensure access to more predictable care.

Under such an approach, the cost of private insurance would be greatly reduced, probably to about 25 to 30 percent of current premium levels. Public coverage up to that amount might be financed through payroll taxes or general revenues. It also might be financed through some form of "premium." While the notion of using premiums may not appear possible since the program is publicly financed, if the program were administered by private companies, they could collect these premiums for the state. If premiums were used, because the public sector is at risk for the basic coverage, the state would be responsible for the costs of coverage that exceeded the total amount of premiums collected. The reason for using all premiums would be to avoid the need to create new taxes explicitly to finance the program, thus making it more politically palatable.

Coverage would not be employer-based, and thus premium levels would not vary across the population. Also, these premiums might be subsidized for low-income and unemployed individuals. Clearly, the payroll tax might obviate the need for such explicit subsidies.

The basic benefit package would emphasize access to preventive and primary services and define a minimum level of coverage to which all people would be entitled. The private, catastrophic coverage would be consistent with that defined package, and would be purchased through the employer, community-rated, and subsidized, possibly through Medicaid, for those unable to afford even this level of coverage.

What are the reasons for considering this approach? Principally because it assigns the most appropriate roles to the public and private sectors. Basic coverage, including preventive services, is problematic from the perspective of insurance. Catastrophic coverage may be a more appropriate role for private insurers to play. It also would permit insurers to continue to compete on the basis of both their catastrophic plans and supplementary packages, as well as on contracts to administer the program. Further, as with the other approaches, it would ensure universal coverage. Finally, since the state would be the primary payor for all people, this approach would permit the kind of leverage over the system and the uniformity necessary to reduce costs.

However, this approach does represent a shift from the current system and would require considerable exploration to define the respective roles. For example, what level of coverage should be considered basic? How should that level increase over time? How should the financing be done? What would be the respective roles of the private insurers and the state in containing costs?

Given that for most people net health insurance costs would not increase—and would possibly decrease—and that publicly financing basic health care could remedy many of the problems with the current system, further consideration is merited.

What Can Governors Do Now?

All three reform approaches represent a continuum of choices ranging from modest incremental change to significant restructuring of the system. While they fall along that continuum, they are not mutually exclusive. In many cases, they are mutually dependent. For example, regardless of how the system is financed, insurance market reform and increased uniformity across all payors might be vital.

In addition, as a state moves along the continuum, the need for greater knowledge increases. Demonstrations are a way to gain this knowledge. Experimentation will require a more cooperative effort between the private and public sectors, as well as more flexibility with respect to federal programs and policy.

The current system does not serve the best interests of anyone. Costs—both public and private—are out of control. And despite the $700 billion the nation spends on health care each year, many Americans are deprived of access to needed services. While providers now maintain some level of adequate reimbursement, that also is eroding, and the amount of regulation is growing and progressively denying physicians and other providers discretion over how they practice medicine.

Some fear that changing the system will make things worse. In fact, a more efficient system may be able to provide universal access without added costs and with less microregulation. Reform should not be feared; indeed, the challenges represent an exciting opportunity for all those in the system.

If health care systems are a reflection of societal values, it is time to make the U.S. system reflect the generosity and caring that are so intrinsic to the nation's history and values. Through innovation and experimentation, Governors can seize the opportunity to develop a financing and service delivery system that provides access to all at affordable prices.

References

A. Foster Higgins and Co., Inc. *Health Care Benefits Survey 1990*. Princeton, N.J.: A. Foster Higgins and Co., Inc., 1990.

Alpha Center. *The Deregulation of Services from CON Review*. Prepared for the Maryland Department of Health and Mental Hygiene, July 1985.

Alpha Center. *Study of Maine's CON Program: Final Report*. Prepared for the Maine Bureau of Medical Services, April 1987.

American Hospital Association. *Annual Survey of Hospitals, 1989-90*. Chicago, Ill.: American Hospital Association, 1990.

American Hospital Association, Special Committee on Care for the Indigent. *Cost and Comparison: Recommendations for Avoiding a Crisis in Care for the Medically Indigent*. Chicago, Ill.: American Hospital Association, 1986.

Andersen, R., et al. *Ambulatory Care and Insurance Coverage in an Era of Constraint*. Chicago, Ill.: Pluribus Press, 1987.

Andersen, R., M. Chen, L. Aday, L. Cornelius. "Health Status and Medical Care Utilization." *Health Affairs*, vol. 6, no. 1 (1987), pp. 136-156.

Arthur D. Little, Inc. *Development of an Evaluation Methodology for Use in Assessing Data Available to the Certificate-of-Need (CON) and Health Planning Programs*. Prepared for the U.S. Department of Health and Human Services, Office of the Assistant Secretary for Health (Contract No. 233-79-4003), April 1982.

Arthur D. Little, Inc. *Final Report: A Study of Intermediate Outcomes of the CON Review Process*. Prepared for the U.S. Department of Health and Human Services, Public Health Service, Health Resources Administration, 1982.

Ashby, John L., Jr. "The Impact of Hospital Regulatory Programs on Per Capita Costs, Utilization, and Capital Investment." *Inquiry*, vol. 21, no. 1 (spring 1984).

Barsky, A.J. "The Paradox of Health." *New England Journal of Medicine*, vol. 318, no. 7 (1988), pp. 414-418.

Begley, Charles E., Milton Schoeman, and Herbert Traxler. "Factors That May Explain Interstate Differences in Certificate-of-Need Decisions." *Health Care Financing Review*, 3 (June 1982).

Bovbjerg, R.R., and C. Koller. "State Health Insurance Pools: Current Performance, Future Prospects." *Inquiry*, vol. 23 (summer 1986), pp. 111-121.

Center for Population Options. *School-Based Clinics Enter the '90s: Update, Evaluation, and Future Challenges*. Washington, D.C.: Center for Population Options, 1990.

Centers for Disease Control. "Smoking Attributable Mortality and Years of Potential Life Lost, U.S., 1988." *Mortality and Morbidity Weekly Report*, vol. 40, no. 62.

Chassin, Mark. Presentation to the Florida Task Force on Government Financed Health Care, September 1990.

Cohodes, Donald R. "Interstate Variation in Certificate of Need Programs: A Review and Prospectus." Paper based on *Evaluation of the Effects of Certificate of Need Programs*, by Policy Analysis, Inc., August 1980.

Committee for the Study of the Future of Public Health. *The Future of Public Health*. Washington, D.C.: Institute of Medicine, National Academy of Sciences, 1988.

Congressional Budget Office. *Rising Health Care Costs: Causes, Implications, and Strategies*. Washington, D.C.: U.S. Government Printing Office, April 1991.

Cullum, Howard M. *Draft Report on the Virginia Medical Care Facilities Certificate of Public Need Program*. Richmond, Va.: Virginia Department of Health and Human Resources, October 1990.

Darman, Richard. Director, Office of Management and Budget. *Testimony on the Problem of Rising Health Costs*. Before the U.S. Senate, Finance Committee, April 16, 1991.

Davis et al. "Paying for Preventive Care: Moving the Debate Forward." *American Journal of Preventive Medicine*, vol. 6, no. 4 (1990).

Dunkelberg, John S., Richard W. Furst, and Rodney L. Roenfeldt. "State Rate Review and the Relationship Between Capital Expenditures and Operating Costs." *Inquiry*, vol. 20 (1983).

Eastaugh, Steven R. "Chapter 8: Health Regulation to Constrain Capital Expansion." *Medical Economics and Health Finance*. Boston, Mass.: Auburn House Publishing Company, 1981.

Elixhauser, A. "The Costs of Smoking and the Cost-Effectiveness of Smoking Cessation Programs." *Journal of Public Health Policy*, summer 1980, pp. 218-237.

Employee Benefit Research Institute. "States and Their Role in the U.S. Health Care Delivery System." *Issue Brief*, no. 110 (January 1991).

Farrell, Karen A. *State Expenditure Report*. Washington, D.C.: National Association of State Budget Officers, 1990.

Fine, Jennifer, and Kari E. Super. "Repeal of Some States' CON Laws Spurs Psychiatric Hospital Construction." *Modern Healthcare*, 16 (October 10, 1986).

Finkler, Merton D. "State Rate Setting Revisited." *Health Affairs*, vol. 6, no. 4 (winter 1987).

Foley, Jill D. *Uninsured in the United States: The Nonelderly Population without Health Insurance*. Washington, D.C.: Employee Benefit Research Institute, April 1991.

Ginsberg, Paul B., and Daniel M. Koretz. "Bed Availability and Hospital Utilization: Estimates of the Roemer Effect." *HCFA Review*, fall 1983.

Griss, B. *Access to Health Care*, vol. 1, no. 3. Washington, D.C.: World Institute on Disability, December 1988.

Griss, B. *Access to Health Care*, vol. 1, no. 4. Washington, D.C.: World Institute on Disability, March 1989.

Hadley, Jack, and Katherine Swartz. "The Impacts on Hospital Costs Between 1980 and 1984 of Hospital Rate Regulation, Competition, and Changes in Health Insurance Coverage." *Inquiry*, vol. 26 (spring 1989).

Hadley, J., E.P. Steinberg, and J. Feder. "Comparison of Uninsured and Privately Insured Hospital Patients." *Journal of the American Medical Association*, vol. 265, no. 3 (1991), pp. 374-379.

Haley, Robert W. *Managing Hospital Control for Cost-Effectiveness*. Chicago, Ill.: American Hospital Publishing, Inc., 1986.

Hartzke, Larry. "Reexamining Certificate of Need Review." Madison, Wis.: Institute for Health Planning, April 1982.

Havighurst, Clark C., and Robert S. McDonough. "The Lithotripsy Game in North Carolina: A New Technology Under Regulation and Deregulation." *Indiana Law Review*, vol. 19, no. 4 (1986).

Health Care Financing Administration, Bureau of Data Management and Strategy. HCFA Forms 2082, 1989.

Health Care Financing Administration, Office of the Actuary, Division of National Cost Estimates. "National Health Expenditures, 1986-2000." *HCFA Review*, summer 1987.

Health Care Financing Administration, Office of the Actuary, Division of National Cost Estimates. "National Health Expenditures, 1988." *HCFA Review*, vol. 11, no. 4 (summer 1990).

Health Care Financing Administration, Office of Intergovernmental Affairs. *Medicaid Services by State*. Washington, D.C.: Health Care Financing Administration, 1990.

Health Facilities Commission, State of Tennessee. "Health Care at the Crossroads: A Survey of Certificate of Need Programs in the United States as Compared to Tennessee," January 1990.

Health Insurance Association of America. *The Health Insurance Industry Strategy for Containing Health Care Costs: A Report to the Board of Directors*. Washington, D.C.: Health Insurance Association of America, February 1990.

Health Insurance Association of America. *Mandated Benefits in Health Insurance Policies*. Washington, D.C.: Health Insurance Association of America, February 15, 1991.

Health Insurance Association of America. *Providing Employee Health Benefits: How Firms Differ*. Washington, D.C.: Health Insurance Association of America, January 1990.

Health Insurance Association of America. *Source Book of Health Insurance Data, 1990*. Washington, D.C.: Health Insurance Association of America, 1990.

Heller, Gloria, and Mary Chase. "A Summary of A Study of the Impact of Deregulation on Health Facilities in Arizona." Arizona Department of Health Services, Office Planning and Budget Development, November 1985.

Hellinger, Fred J. "The Effect of Certificate-of-Need Legislation on Hospital Investment." *Inquiry*, vol. 13 (June 1976).

Hendershot, G. "Health Status and Medical Care Utilization." *Health Affairs*, vol. 7, no. 1 (1988), pp. 114-121.

Hershey, Nathan, and Deborah Robinson. "Health Planning and Certificate of Need: The Quality Dimension." *Health Policy Quarterly*, vol. 1, no. 4 (winter 1981).

Hill, Ian, and Janine Breyel. *Caring for Kids*. Washington, D.C.: National Governors' Association, 1991.

Howard, Marcia A. *Fiscal Survey of the States*. Washington, D.C.: National Governors' Association and National Association of State Budget Officers, September 1990.

Howell, Julianne R. "Regulating Hospital Capital Investment: The Experience in Massachusetts," 1984.

Hughes D., et al. *The Health of American Children*. Washington, D.C.: Children's Defense Fund, 1989.

Hurdle, S., and G.C. Pope. "Physician Productivity: Trends and Determinants." *Inquiry*, vol. 26 (1989), pp. 100-115.

Institute of Medicine. *Preventing Low Birthweight*. Washington, D.C.: National Academy Press, 1985.

Intergovernmental Health Policy Project. "States Break Down Malpractice Barriers to Prenatal Care Access." *State Health Notes*, no. 105 (July-August 1990).

Intergovernmental Health Policy Project. "1989 Update: CON Program Changes." *State Health Notes*.

Johnston, William B. *Workforce 2000: Work and Workers for the Twenty-first Century*. Indianapolis, Ind.: Hudson Institute, Inc., June 1987.

Keeler, E.B., et al. "How Free Care Reduced Hypertension in the Health Insurance Experiment." *Journal of the American Medical Association*, vol. 254, no. 14 (1985), pp. 1926-1931.

Kindig, D.A., et al. "Trends in Physician Availability in 10 Urban Areas from 1963 to 1980." *Inquiry*, vol. 24, no. 2 (1987), pp. 136-146.

Kinzer, David. "The Decline and Fall of Deregulation." *New England Journal of Medicine*, 318 (January 14, 1988).

Kristein, M. "The Economics of Health Promotion at the Worksite." *Health Education Quarterly*, vol. 9 (supplement, 1982), pp. 27-36.

Lave, J.R. "Cost Containment Policies in Long-term Care." *Inquiry*, vol. 22 (spring 1985).

Lawthers-Higgins, Ann, Cynthia Taft, and Jane Hodgman. "The Impact of Certificate of Need on CAT Scanning in Massachusetts." *Health Care Management Review*, summer 1984.

Lazenby, Helen C., and Suzanne W. Letsch. "National Health Expenditures, 1989." *Health Care Financing Review*, vol. 12, no. 2 (winter 1990), pp. 1-13.

Levit, Katharine R., and Cathy A. Cowan. "The Burden of Health Care Costs: Business, Households, and Governments." *Health Care Financing Review*, vol. 12, no. 2 (winter 1990), pp. 127-137.

Lewin and Associates, Inc. *Certificate of Need and the Changing Market: An Analysis for the Illinois Health Care Cost Containment Council*, September 15, 1987.

Lewin and Associates, Inc. *The Experience with the Section 1122 Capital Expenditure Review Program*, January 1, 1985.

Lewin/ICF. "Analysis of Proposals Related to Kentucky's Certificate of Need Program." Washington, D.C.: Lewin/ICF, November 15, 1989.

Lewin/ICF. *The Health Care Financing System and the Uninsured*. Washington, D.C.: Lewin/ICF, April 4, 1990.

Lewis-Idema, Deborah. *Factors Influencing Medicaid Reimbursement to Community and Migrant Health Centers*. Washington, D.C.: National Association of Community Health, 1990.

Lewis-Idema, Deborah. *Increasing Provider Participation: Strategies for Improving State Perinatal Programs*. Washington, D.C.: National Governors' Association, July 1988.

Martin E. Segal Company. "Rise in State Employee Health Plan Costs Moderates: Survey of State Employee Health Benefit Plans, Summary of Findings." New York, N.Y.: Martin E. Segal Company, 1990.

Mayo, John W., and Deborah A. McFarland. "Regulation, Market Structure, and Hospital Costs." *Southern Economic Journal*, 55 (January 1989).

McCloskey, Amanda, and John Luehrs. *State Initiatives to Improve Rural Health Care*. Washington, D.C.: National Governors' Association, 1990.

Melnick, G., J. Mann, and C. Serrato. *Hospital Costs and Patient Access Under the New Jersey Hospital Rate-Setting System*. Santa Monica, Calif.: RAND Corporation, September 1988.

Melnick, Glenn A., and Jack Zwanziger. "Hospital Behavior Under Competition and Cost-Containment Policies: The California Experience, 1980 to 1985." *Journal of the American Medical Association*, vol. 260, no. 18 (November 11, 1988).

Merrill, Jeffrey C. *State Initiatives for the Medically Uninsured*, Annual Supplement, HCFA Publication No. 03311. Washington, D.C.: U.S. Government Printing Office, December 1990.

Merrill, Jeffrey, and Catherine McLaughlin. "Competition Versus Regulation: Some Empirical Evidence." *Journal of Health Politics, Policy, and Law*, 10 (winter 1986).

Mine Diabetes Control Project. "Impact of Diabetes Outpatient Education Program." *Morbidity and Mortality Weekly Report*, vol. 31, no. 23 (1982), pp. 307-314.

National Governors' Association. *Catalogue of State Medicaid Program Changes*. Washington, D.C.: National Governors' Association, 1990.

National Governors' Association. "State Coverage of Pregnant Women and Children." *MCH Update*. Washington, D.C.: National Governors' Association, January 1991.

National Leadership Commission on Health Care. *For the Health of a Nation: A Shared Responsibility*. Ann Arbor, Mich.: Health Administration Press, 1989.

Needleman, Jack, Judith Arnold, John Sheils, and Lawrence S. Lewin. *The Health Care Financing System and the Uninsured*. Washington, D.C.: Lewin/ICF, 1990.

"New Worries About Old Diseases." *Newsweek*, May 27, 1991.

Newacheck, P.W., and B. Starfield. "Morbidity and Use of Ambulatory Care Services among Poor Children." *American Journal of Public Health*, vol. 78, no. 8 (1988), pp. 927-933.

Nyman, John. "Excess Demand, Consumer Rationality, and the Quality of Care in Regulated Nursing Homes." *Health Services Research*, April 1989.

Pauly, M.V., and P. Wilson. "Hospital Output Forecasts and the Cost of Empty Hospital Beds." Health Services Research, August 1986.

The Pepper Commission, U.S. Bipartisan Commission on Comprehensive Health Care. *A Call for Action*. Washington, D.C.: U.S. Government Printing Office, September 1990.

Policy Analysis, Inc., and Urban Systems Research and Engineering, Inc. "Evaluation of the Effects of Certificate of Need Programs. Volume 1: Executive Summary." Prepared for the Health Resources Service Administration, January 1981.

Reider, Alan E., John R. Mason, and Leonard H. Glantz. "Certificate of Need: The Massachusetts Experience." *American Journal of Law and Medicine*, vol. 1, no. 1 (March 1975).

Robinson, James C., Deborah W. Garnick, and Stephen J. McPhee. "Market and Regulatory Influences on the Availability of Coronary Angioplasty and Bypass Surgery in U.S. Hospitals." *New England Journal of Medicine*, July 9, 1987.

Robinson, James C., and Harold S. Luft. "Competition, Regulation, and Hospital Costs, 1982 to 1986." *Journal of the American Medical Association*, November 11, 1988.

Roemer, Milton, and Max Shain. *Hospital Utilization Under Insurance*. Chicago, Ill.: American Hospital Association, 1959.

Rosenbaum, Sara, and Dana Hughes. "Appendix C: The Medical Malpractice Crisis and Poor Women." In *Prenatal Care: Reaching Mothers, Reaching Infants*. Washington, D.C.: National Academy Press, 1988.

Salkever, David S., and Thomas W. Bice. *Milbank Memorial Fund Quarterly*, spring 1976.

Scanlon, William J. "A Theory of the Nursing Home Market." *Inquiry*, spring 1980.

Scanlon, William, and Judith Feder. "Regulation of Investment in Long-term Care Facilities." *Intentions and Consequences of Regulating the Nursing Home Bed Supply*. Working Paper 1218-9. Washington, D.C.: The Urban Institute, January 1980.

Schneider, Don. "Economic Impact and Project Selection Methodology for Certificate of Need." Final report submitted to the New York State Health Planning Commission, 1980.

Schramm, C.J., S.C. Renn, and B. Biles. "New Perspectives on State Rate Setting." *Health Affairs*, fall 1986.

Schwartz, William B. "The Regulation Strategy for Controlling Hospital Cost: Problems and Prospects." *New England Journal of Medicine*, November 19, 1981.

Schwartz, W.B., and P.L. Joskow. "Duplicated Hospital Facilities: How Much Can We Save By Consolidating Them?" *New England Journal of Medicine*, December 18, 1980.

Schwartz, W.B., and D.N. Mendelson. "No Evidence of an Emerging Physician Surplus: An Analysis of Change in Physicians' Work Load and Income." *Journal of the American Medical Association*, January 26, 1990.

Sloan, Frank A., and Randall R. Bovbjerg. *Medical Malpractice: Crisis, Response and Effects*. Research Bulletin. Washington D.C.: Health Insurance Association of America, May 1989.

Sloan, F.A., D.M. Mergenhagen, and R.R. Bovbjerg. "Effects of Tort Reforms on the Value of Closed Medical Malpractice Claims: A Microanaylsis." *Journal of Health Politics, Policy and Law*, winter 1989.

Sloan, F.A., and W.B. Schwartz. "More Doctors: What Will They Cost?" *Journal of the American Medical Association*, 1983.

Sloan, Frank A., and Bruce Steinwald. "Effects of Regulation on Hospital Costs and Input Use." *Journal of Law and Economics*, April 1980.

Sloan, Frank A., Joseph Valvona, James M. Perrin, and Killard W. Adamache. "Diffusion of Surgical Technology: An Exploratory Study." *Journal of Health Economics*, 1986.

Smeeding, T.M. *Measuring and Valuing the Economic Benefits of Diabetes Control: The Economic Perspective*. Salt Lake City, Utah: University of Utah, Department of Economics, April 1983.

Starr, Paul. *The Social Transformation of American Medicine*. New York: Basic Books, 1982.

Steinwald, Bruce, and Frank A. Sloan. "Regulatory Approaches to Hospital Cost Containment: A Synthesis of the Empirical Evidence." *A New Approach to the Economics of Health Care*, edited by M. Olson. Washington, D.C.: American Enterprise Institute, 1981.

Stewart, Charles. White paper on the effects of CON on the health care industry in Alabama. Alabama State Health Planning and Development Agency, September 1988.

Stiles, Samuel V. *Briefing Paper on Certificate of Need*. Alpha Center, February 1983.

Swartz, Katherine. "Why Requiring Employers to Provide Health Insurance Is a Bad Idea." *Journal of Health Politics, Policy, and Law*, vol. 15, no. 4 (winter 1990).

U.S. Congress, Office of Technology Assessment. *Health Care in Rural America*. Washington, D.C.: Office of Technology Assessment, September 1990.

U.S. Department of Commerce, Bureau of the Census. *Statistical Abstract of the United States: 1990*. Washington, D.C.: U.S. Department of Commerce, 1991.

U.S. Department of Health and Human Services, National Center for Health Services Research. "Research on Competition in the Financing and Delivery of Health Services: A Summary of Policy Issues." DHHS Pub. No. (PHS) 83-3328-1, 1982.

U.S. Department of Health and Human Services, Public Health Service. *Healthy People 2000*. Washington, D.C.: U.S. Department of Health and Human Services, 1990.

U.S. Department of Labor, Bureau of Labor Statistics. *Employer Benefits in Medium and Large Firms*. Washington, D.C.: U.S. Government Printing Office, 1988.

U.S. General Accounting Office. *Canadian Health Insurance: Lessons for the United States*. Washington, D.C.: U.S. General Accounting Office, June 1991.

U.S. General Accounting Office. *Workers At Risk: Increased Number in Contingent Employment Lack Insurance, Other Benefits*. Washington, D.C.: U.S. General Accounting Office, March 1991.

U.S. House of Representatives, Committee on Ways and Means. *Overview of Entitlement Programs: 1991 Green Book*. Washington, D.C.: U.S. Government Printing Office, May 7, 1991.

U.S. Preventive Services Task Force. *Guide to Clinical Preventive Services: An Assessment of the Effectiveness of 169 Interventions*. Baltimore, Md.: Williams and Wilkins, 1989.

Waldo, David R., Sally T. Sonnefiled, David McKusick, and Ross H. Arnett III. "Health Expenditures by Age Group, 1977 and 1987." *HCFA Review*, summer 1989.

Washington State Health Care Authority. "Study of State Purchased Health Care." Olympia, Wash.: Washington State Health Care Authority, December 1990.

White, C.C., J.P. Koplan, and W.A. Orenstein. "Benefits, Risks, and Costs of Immunizations for Measles, Mumps, and Rubella." *American Journal of Public Health*, vol. 75, no. 7 (1985), pp. 739-744.

Wickizer, Thomas M., John R.C. Wheeler, and Paul J. Feldstein. "Does Utilization Review Reduce Unnecessary Hospital Care and Contain Costs?" *Medical Care*, June 1989.

Wilensky, G. "Health Care, the Poor, and the Role of Medicaid." *Health Affairs*, vol. 1, no. 4 (1982), pp. 93-100.

Woolhandler, S., and D. U. Himmelstein. "The Deteriorating Administrative Efficiency of the U.S. Health Care System." *New England Journal of Medicine*, vol. 324, no. 18, pp. 1253-1258.

Woolhandler, S., and D.U. Himmelstein. "Reverse Targeting of Preventive Care Due to Lack of Health Insurance." *Journal of the American Medical Association*, vol. 259 (1988), pp. 2872-2874.

Regional Hearings on Potential State Strategies for Health Care Reform

HEALTH CARE COST CONTAINMENT STRATEGIES

Wilmington, Delaware, June 17, 1991
Governor Michael N. Castle, Delaware

Governor Michael N. Castle of Delaware, co-vice-chair of the National Governors' Association's Task Force on Health Care, led a regional field hearing focused on cost containment strategies. Four panels of health care providers, insurance providers, private sector representatives, and public sector representatives discussed practices through which escalating health care costs can be contained. The majority of approaches discussed focused on cost containment practices that are viable within the existing health insurance system.

Health Care Providers

Ali Z. Hameli, M.D.
President, Medical Society of Delaware

Allen Johnson
Delaware Hospital Association

Donald T. Lewers, M.D., FACP
American Medical Association

Andrea Scharf
Executive Director, Pennsylvania Association of Health Maintenance Organizations

Yrene Waldron
Director of Admissions and Public Relations, Leader Nursing and Rehabilitation Center

Insurance Providers

Paul P. Cooper III
Vice President of Health Care Policy, The Prudential

Jim Meehan
Assistant General Counsel
Connecticut General of North America

Marshall Rozzi
Executive Vice President, U.S. Health Care

Robert E. Tremain
Senior Vice President of Health Care, Blue Cross and Blue Shield of Delaware, Inc.

Elliot Wicks
Associate Director for Policy Studies, Health Insurance Association of America

Private Sector

Terrence M. Adlhock
Counsel, Southern California Edison

Steven Harrison
Director of Compensation and Benefits, The DuPont Company

Jim Williams
Group Manager of Health Coalitions, GLAXO, Inc.

Stephen P. Woods
Vice President, National Federation of Independent Business

Public Sector

Jack H. Boger
National Legislative Council, American Association of Retired Persons

Gerry Goodrich
Deputy Commissioner of Health, New Jersey Department of Health

Muriel Rusten
Deputy Secretary, Delaware Department of Health and Social Services

Nelson Sabatini
Secretary, Maryland Department of Health and Mental Hygiene

ACCESS TO PRIMARY AND PREVENTIVE CARE

Little Rock, Arkansas, June 19, 1991
Governor Bill Clinton, Arkansas

Governor Bill Clinton of Arkansas, co-vice-chair of the National Governors' Association's Task Force on Health Care, hosted a regional field hearing that explored ways to improve access to primary and preventive health care. The hearing addressed three areas of concern in primary and preventive care: pregnant women and young children, school-age children and adolescents, and adults and the elderly. Common needs experienced by all three groups are increased health education to assist in fostering healthier lifestyles and improved access to health care services.

Panel One: Pregnant Women and Young Children

Antoinette Eaton, M.D.
President, American Academy of Pediatrics
Columbus, Ohio

Shelly Gehshan
Deputy Director, Southern Regional Project on Infant
Mortality, Washington, D.C.

David Adams
Administrator, Health Services, Sunbeam Appliance
Company, Coushapta, Louisiana

Earl and Mary Belle
Home Instruction Program for Preschool Youngsters
(HIPPY), Pearcy, Arkansas

Bettye Caldwell
Donghey Distinguished Professor of Education, Center for
Child Development, University of Arkansas at Little Rock

Jackie Horton
Director, Division of Minority Health
Missouri Department of Health

Panel Two: School-Age Children and Adolescents

Joycelyn Elders, M.D.
Director, Arkansas Department of Health

Dianne O'Connor, R.N.,
W.A. Perry Middle School, Columbia, South Carolina

Amy Rossi
Executive Director, Arkansas Advocates for Children and
Families, Little Rock, Arkansas

Kirk Thompson
High School Senior, McClellan High School
Little Rock, Arkansas

Frankie Sarver
Executive Director, Fighting Back Project
Little Rock, Arkansas

Panel Three: Adults and the Elderly

Leona Young, R.N.
Executive Director, Morton Comprehensive Health
Services, Inc., Tulsa, Oklahoma

Dan Schulder
Legislative Director, National Council of Citizens
Washington, D.C.

David Tennenbaum
Blue Cross and Blue Shield Association, Chicago, Illinois

Henry McHenry
Regional Vice President, National Alliance of Business
Dallas, Texas

Cecil Malone
Arkansas State Director, American Association of Retired
Persons, Little Rock, Arkansas

Respondents

J. Edward Hill, M.D.
American Medical Association's Council on Legislation
Hollandale, Mississippi

Sarah Shuptrine
President, Shuptrine and Associates
Columbia, South Carolina

Walter Shepherd, M.D.
Executive Director, Governor's Commission on Reduction
of Infant Mortality, Raleigh, North Carolina

Buddy Menn
Assistant to Counsel, Health Insurance Association of
America, Washington, D.C.

Rural Health Care Strategies

Sioux Falls, South Dakota, June 20, 1991

Governor George S. Mickelson, South Dakota

Governor Arne H. Carlson, Minnesota

Governor George A. Sinner, North Dakota

Governor George S. Mickelson of South Dakota chaired a regional field hearing that focused on strategies to improve rural health care. Governor Arne H. Carlson of Minnesota and Governor George A. Sinner of North Dakota also participated in the session. Panelists said that states and rural communities would be able to develop better networking arrangements if they had more freedom to experiment with new or alternative models of care as replications of urban health care models do not work in the majority of rural areas. Governor Mickelson added that both innovation and flexibility are prerequisites to a viable rural health care system.

Health Professionals Panelists

Donald L. Weaver, M.D.
Director, National Health Service Corps
Rockville, Maryland

Gerald C. Keller, M.D.
Chairman, Rural Health Task Force
American Academy of Family Physicians
Manville, Louisiana

David N. Sundwall, M.D.
Chairman, National Advisory, Council Health Professions
Education, Washington, D.C.

Thomas M. Dean, M.D.
Immediate Past President, National Rural Health
Association, Wessington Springs, South Dakota

Charles North, M.D.
Senior Clinician for Family Practice, Public Health Service
Indian Hospital, Albuquerque, New Mexico

Jean Thompson, FNP, PA-C
Clinical Director, East River Health Care, Inc.
Howard, South Dakota

Health Programs Panelists

Jeffrey Human
Director, Office of Rural Health Policy, Rockville, Maryland

Fred Moskol
President, National Rural Health Association
Madison, Wisconsin

Christopher Atchison
Director, Iowa Department of Public Health
Des Moines, Iowa

Peter Maningas, M.D.
Chairman, Rural Emergency Medical Services Committee
National Association of Emergency Medical Services
Physicians, Rapid City, South Dakota

Audrey Nora, M.D., M.P.H.
Assistant Surgeon General, Regional Health Administrator
Region VIII, Denver, Colorado

Health Facilities Panelists

Tom Cherry
Director, Montana Hospital Research and Education
Foundation, Helena, Montana

Gale Walker
Administrator, St. Michael's Hospital
Tyndall, South Dakota

Darryl Leong, M.D., M.P.H.
Director of Clinic Affairs, National Association of
Community Health Centers, Washington, D.C.

Andrea Walsh
Assistant Commissioner, Bureau of Health Resources and
Managed Care, Minnesota Department of Health

William R. Taylor, M.D.
South Dakota State Senator, Aberdeen, South Dakota

INSURANCE REFORM AND SMALL MARKET REFORM

Vancouver, Washington, June 25, 1991
Governor Booth Gardner, Washington

Governor Booth Gardner of Washington, chairman of the National Governors' Association and of the Task Force on Health Care, led a regional field hearing that explored the role of health insurers in the health care system and the problems small businesses face in purchasing affordable health insurance for their employees. Participants indicated that all involved in health care are dissatisfied with the existing U.S. system. Small businesses are the most dissatisfied with the employer-based system. Participants warned that if steps are not taken to control health care costs, more and more people will be denied access. Furthermore, health care expenses will claim an even larger share of state revenues—resources that otherwise could be invested in education, public safety, and the environment.

Roundtable Participants

Andrea Castell
Executive Director, Health Care Purchasers Association of South Sound , Seattle, Washington

Jack Lewin
Director, Hawaii Department of Health

Ron Lewis
Proprietor, Greenwood True Value Hardware
Seattle, Washington

Ed Nieubuurt
Chair, Oregon Insurance Pool Governing Board
Portland, Oregon

Donald P. Sacco
President and CEO, Pierce County Medical
Tacoma, Washington

Richard Seaman, M.D.
Vice President, Washington State Medical Association
Olympia, Washington

Jeff Selberg
Administrator, Southwest Washington Medical Center
Vancouver, Washington

Gubernatorial Representatives

Winston Barton
Office of the Governor, Oklahoma City, Oklahoma

George J. Neumayer
Acting Director, Department of Insurance, Boise, Idaho

Panel One

The Honorable Peter Brooks, M.D.
Advisory Council, Washington Basic Health Plan
Walla Walla, Washington

Sylvia Beck
Executive Director, Washington State Board of Health

Ruth Scarborough
National Association of Retired Persons
Vancouver, Washington

Panel Two

Gary L. Smith
Independent Business Association, Bellevue, Washington

Rick Curtis
Director, Policy Development and Research Health
Insurance Association of America, Washington, D.C.

Gretchen Babcock
Executive Director, State Services
Blue Cross and Blue Shield Association, Washington, D.C.

John Hartnedy
Vice President and Actuary
Golden Rule Insurance Company of Illinois

Scott Hass
Oregon & Washington Association of Health Underwriters
Portland, Oregon

Panel Three

Tom Milne
Southwest Washington Health District
Vancouver, Washington

Kamala Bremer
Human Services Council, Vancouver, Washington

Patti Robertson, R.N.
Holland Associates, Gig Harbor, Washington

Leslie Woodruff
Woodruff Company & Community Health Care
Association, West Seattle, Washington

Frank Morris
Puget Sound Council of Senior Citizens, Washington State
Retired Teachers' Association, Seattle, Washington

Acknowledgements

The Task Force on Health Care of the National Governors' Association provided the leadership and guidance for this report. The task force was chaired by Governor Booth Gardner of Washington, and Governor Bill Clinton of Arkansas and Governor Michael N. Castle of Delaware served as vice chairs. Other task force Governors involved in the development of the report include Pete Wilson of California, Lowell P. Weicker Jr. of Connecticut, Lawton Chiles of Florida, John Waihee of Hawaii, Jim Edgar of Illinois, Terry E. Branstad of Iowa, Buddy Roemer of Louisiana, John R. McKernan Jr. of Maine, John Engler of Michigan, John Ashcroft of Missouri, Jim Florio of New Jersey, Carroll A. Campbell Jr. of South Carolina, and Ann W. Richards of Texas.

Former task force Governors who made substantial contributions in the early stages of the report include Michael S. Dukakis of Massachusetts, James J. Blanchard of Michigan, Garrey E. Carruthers of New Mexico, Richard F. Celeste of Ohio, and Edward D. DiPrete of Rhode Island.

Governors Arne H. Carlson of Minnesota, Bob Miller of Nevada, George A. Sinner of North Dakota, and George S. Mickelson of South Dakota also provided substantial guidance on various sections of the report.

The National Governors' Association acknowledges the generous financial support of the Pew Charitable Trusts for this project.

Many people contributed to the development of this report. Thanks are due to the members of the Health Care Task Force Staff Advisory Council, whose guidance was invaluable: Robert Crittenden (Washington), Carol Rasco (Arkansas), Kathryn Way (Delaware), Stan Marshburn (Washington), Stephanie Solien (Washington), S. Kimberly Belshe (California), Ben Haddad (California), Jan Kaplan (Connecticut), Terry Muilenburg (Connecticut), Martha Naismith (Florida), Gary Clarke (Florida), Peter Sybinsky (Hawaii), Janice Lipsen (Hawaii), Phil Shimer (Hawaii), Kate Sullivan (Illinois), Phil Smith (Iowa), James Burns (Louisiana), Elizabeth Beard (Louisiana), Lisa Lacasse (Maine), Rich Silkman (Maine), LeAnne Redick (Michigan), Dennis Shornack (Michigan), Gerald H. Miller (Michigan), Marise Stewart (Missouri), Charlie Stokes (Missouri), Linda Hillemann (Missouri), Missy Shaffer (New Jersey), Nikki McNamee (South Carolina), Jim Bradford (South Carolina), Margaret Key (South Carolina), Barbara Smith (South Dakota), Pat Cole (Texas), and Bridgette Taylor (Texas).

Former members of the task force staff who assisted with the report include Mike Nardone (Massachusetts), Kris Balderston (Massachusetts), Maura Cullen (Michigan), Patience Drake (Michigan), Gary Granere (New Mexico), Ann Toch (Ohio), and Robert Comiskey (Rhode Island).

Appreciation is also due to the following consultants who wrote chapters, provided expert assistance, or reviewed drafts of the report: Stuart Altman, Robert J. Blendon, Patricia Butler, Timothy Eckels, Jennifer Edwards, Lynn Etheredge, Judy Feder, Barbara Matula, Deborah A. McFarland, Jeffrey C. Merrill, Jack Needleman, Richard Saltman, and John Sheils.

Among the National Governors' Association staff who contributed to this project are Raymond C. Scheppach, Alicia Pelrine, John Luehrs, Janine Breyel, Stephanie Cook-Hall, Ann Danelski, Amanda McCloskey, Kathleen Miller, Barbara Tymann, and L. Carl Volpe. Karen Glass of the NGA Office of Public Affairs edited the manuscript and Rae Young Bond, Gerry Feinstein, and Mark Miller provided editorial assistance.